Handbook of Forensic Nursing

Handbook of Forensic Nursing

Suresh K. Sharma, PhD, RN, FNRS
Professor & Principal
College of Nursing
All India Institute of Medical Sciences
Jodhpur, Rajasthan

Tanuj Kanchan, MD, MAMS, FIAMLE, FIALFS
Dean (Research)
Professor & Head
Department of Forensic Medicine & Toxicology
All India Institute of Medical Sciences
Jodhpur, Rajasthan

ELSEVIER

ELSEVIER

RELX India Pvt. Ltd.
Registered Office: 818, Indraprakash Building, 21, Barakhamba Road, New Delhi 110 001
Corporate Office: 14th Floor, Building No. 10B, DLF Cyber City, Phase II, Gurgaon-122 002, Haryana, India

Handbook of Forensic Nursing, Suresh K. Sharma and Tanuj Kanchan

ISBN: 978-81-312-6640-3
e-ISBN: 978-81-312-6641-0
ISBN: 978-81-312-6723-3 (Set)
e-Book ISBN: 978-81-312-6724-0 (Set)
This book is part of the set ISBN: 978-81-312-6723-3. Not to be sold separately.

First Printed in India 2023, Reprinted 2024

Notice

Content Strategist: Deepti Damodaran
Content Project Manager: Subodh Kumar
Sr Cover Designer: Milind Majgaonkar
Sr Production Executive: Dhan Singh Rana

Printed at Rajkamal Electric Press, Kundli, Haryana.

PREFACE

Forensic nursing is an emerging field that plays a crucial role at the intersection of health care and the legal system. It combines the specialized knowledge and skills of nursing with an understanding of the legal principles and processes. In recent years, forensic nursing has gained recognition worldwide as an essential discipline in addressing the complex health care needs of individuals involved in legal matters.

In context of India, the field of forensic nursing is still in its nascent stages. However, given the diverse legal landscape and the growing importance of health care in the country, the need for well-trained forensic nurses is becoming increasingly apparent. These professionals are equipped to provide comprehensive care to victims of violence, collect and preserve evidence, and contribute to the effective administration of justice.

The *Handbook of Forensic Nursing* aims to bridge the existing gap by providing a comprehensive resource for forensic nurses, health care practitioners, legal professionals and law enforcement agencies in India. This handbook serves as a valuable tool in understanding the role of forensic nursing within the Indian legal framework and how it contributes to the overall justice system.

This handbook is divided into five units that cover various aspects of forensic nursing practice in India. It begins with an introduction to the field, discussing the historical development of forensic nursing and its current relevance in the Indian context. The subsequent chapters delve into the legal aspects of forensic nursing, examining the relevant Indian laws, regulations and guidelines that govern the practice.

The handbook also explores the different types of forensic nursing, such as sexual assault examination, domestic violence assessment, child abuse evaluation and Indian judicial system. Each section provides a detailed overview of the specific skills, techniques and protocols required for effective practice.

Moreover, the handbook emphasizes the importance of interdisciplinary collaboration, highlighting the critical partnerships between forensic nurses, health care professionals, legal experts and law enforcement agencies. It recognizes the need for cohesive teamwork to ensure a seamless integration of forensic nursing into the broader legal and health care systems.

Furthermore, this handbook incorporates practical examples and ethical considerations to enhance the reader's understanding and application of forensic nursing principles. It provides guidance on best practices, evidence collection, documentation and courtroom testimony, enabling forensic nurses to contribute effectively as expert witnesses.

The *Handbook of Forensic Nursing* is a culmination of the collective expertise and experiences of renowned forensic nursing professionals, and forensic and medical jurisprudence experts in India. It is a valuable resource that aims to empower forensic nurses, facilitate knowledge exchange and foster the growth of this specialized field within the Indian health care and legal systems.

We hope that this handbook serves as a foundation for promoting excellence in forensic nursing practice, protecting the rights of victims, and upholding the principles of justice in India. By equipping forensic nurses with the necessary knowledge and skills, we can pave the way for a more comprehensive, compassionate and effective response to the health care needs of individuals involved in legal matters.

Suresh K. Sharma
Tanuj Kanchan

CONTRIBUTORS

1. Tanuj Kanchan, Dean (Research), Professor & Head, Department of Forensic & Toxicology, All India Institute of Medical Sciences, Jodhpur, Rajasthan
2. Vikash P. Meshram, Associate Professor, Department of Forensic & Toxicology, All India Institute of Medical Sciences, Jodhpur, Rajasthan
3. Nipin Kalal, Assistant Professor, College of Nursing, All India Institute of Medical Sciences, Jodhpur, Rajasthan
4. Nancy Kurian, Tutor, College of Nursing, All India Institute of Medical Sciences, Jodhpur, Rajasthan
5. Joyce Joseph, Lecturer, College of Nursing, All India Institute of Medical Sciences, Raipur, Chhattisgarh
6. Hemlata, Tutor, College of Nursing, All India Institute of Medical Sciences, Jodhpur, Rajasthan
7. Jaison Joseph, Assistant Lecturer, College of Nursing, Pt. B.D. Sharma University of Health Sciences, Rohtak, Haryana
8. Sonali Banerjee, Fertility Counsellor, Yoga & Wellness Mentor, Mumbai, Maharashtra
9. Suresh Sharma, Professor & Principal, College of Nursing, All India Institute of Medical Sciences, Jodhpur, Rajasthan

REVIEWERS

1. Sanjeev Lalwani, Professor, Department of Forensic Medicine & Toxicology, and Registrar, AIIMS, New Delhi
2. Rakesh Gorea, Professor & Head, Department of Forensic Medicine and Toxicology, Gian Sagar Medical College and Hospital, Banur, Patiala, Punjab
3. Krishnadutt Chavali, Professor & Head, Department of Department of Forensic Medicine and Toxicology, AIIMS, Raipur, Chattisgarh
4. Binya Bastia, Professor & Head, Department of Forensic Medicine and Toxicology, AIIMS, Rishikesh, Uttarakhand
5. S.J. Nalini, Principal, Professor & Principal, Faculty of Nursing, Sri Ramachandra Institute of Higher Education and Research, Chennai, Tamil Nadu
6. Sukhpal Kaur, Professor & Principal (Actg), National Institute of Nursing Education, PGIMER, Chandigarh
7. Ashok Kumar Bishnoi, Professor & Dean (Nursing), Atal Bihari Medical University, Lucknow, Uttar Pradesh
8. Laxmi Ramamoorthy, Assistant Professor, College of Nursing, JIPMER, Puducherry
9. Shiv Kumar Mudgal, Associate Professor, College of Nursing, AIIMS, Deoghar, Jharkhand

CONTENTS

UNIT

FORENSIC SCIENCE

I

Nancy Kurien and Joyce Joseph

Learning objectives

On completion of this chapter, the readers will be able to:

1. Define forensic science, forensic medicine and forensic nursing.
2. Discuss history of forensic science.
3. Appraise the importance of forensic science in medical science.
4. Discuss meaning, epidemiology and types of violence.
5. Explain risk factors, hazards and preventive strategies of child and woman sexual abuse.

Forensic science

Introduction

In the judicial system, forensic science plays a mounting and crucial role. It generally underpins criminal and civil investigations, and also dispenses expert opinion and scientific details to assist courts in their decisions. That is, forensic science deals with the factual and legal characteristics of an instance. The word, forensic, is derived from the Latin word *forensis* meaning 'public' or 'in open court' or 'of or before the forum'. In ancient times, criminal charges were presented before a group of public in the forum. This might be the reason for suggesting the word *forensic,* meaning '*of or used in courts of law*'. Forensic is a science that deals with the application of scientific knowledge to legal problems. Forensic science is also known as *criminalistics,* as it involves the collection, analysis and interpretation of physical evidence produced by criminal activity. Hans Gross, a researcher in criminal law and procedure, coined the term *kriminalistik.*

Definitions

The term *forensic science* refers to a group of scientific disciplines which are concerned with the application of their particular scientific area of expertise to law enforcement, criminal, civil, legal and judicial matters. Forensic science includes all branches of science and applies scientific techniques to the purpose of the law. All the techniques used in this science were borrowed from various scientific disciplines such as chemistry, medicine, biology and photography.

- The simplest definition of forensic science is *any science that is used for the law or any science that is used within the criminal justice system.*

- Forensic science is the application of scientific knowledge to the definition and enforcement of laws.

History of forensic science

- The use of science in criminal investigations has been documented in the literature before the Roman Empire.
- The first officially recorded autopsy was done by the Roman physician Antisius in 44 BCE, on the corpse of the Roman statesman Julius Caesar.
- The Egyptians, in 3000 BCE, practiced separating and examining the internal organs of humans after death, which is an early example of an autopsy.
- Roman lawyer Quintilian used basic forensics to release an innocent in the 1st century CE.
- The book Xi Yuan Lu by Song Ci (13th century) in China became the earliest accessible literature that helped to determine the threats to life.
- In the 16th century, Italian surgeons Fortunato Fidelis and Paolo Zacchia laid the foundation of modern pathology which studies the changes in the anatomy of the body due to an ailment.
- In 1773, Swedish chemist Carl Wilhelm Scheele first developed a chemical test to detect arsenic in corpses.
- During the 1800s, the application of scientific principles to criminal investigations accelerated. Clothing and vegetable grains could be used to place suspects at the scenes of crimes. The invention of the camera led to the use of photography to document and preserve crime scenes. Hydrogen peroxide was discovered to foam as it oxidized when it contacted haemoglobin. This demonstrated the ability to test for the presence of blood and was considered seminal in the study of serology.
- In 1814, Mathieu Orfila, known as the father of Forensic Toxicology, published the first scientific treatise on the detection of poison.
- Henry Goddard was the foremost to connect a bullet to a weapon (1835).
- In 1880, Sir Francis Galton developed the first technique of fingerprint matching.
- The independent works of Englishmen William Herschel (1738–1822) and Henry Faulds (1843–1930) and American scientist Thomas Taylor (1820–1910) detailed the uniqueness of human fingerprints and their potential use in identifying people led to the codification and standardization of accepted practices within forensic science.
- In 1896, Sir Edward Henry developed the Henry Classification System which was adopted as the standard for criminal fingerprinting techniques around the world.
- Until the mid-19th century, the use of science in investigations was discussed, but the appropriate application of scientific principles had not yet been fully implemented.
- Dr Edmond Locard (1877–1966), a French scientist and criminologist who had studied law and medicine, proposed the notion that 'everything leaves a trace', a principle that prevails today in crime scene investigation. In 1910, Locard drew up the fundamental principles of criminology: 'Every contact retains a clue'. He was called the Sherlock Holmes of France.
- The advancements of the 20th century were built largely upon the groundwork laid in the 19th century, refining techniques in the collection of and preservation of evidence and DNA analysis.
- Recently, the emergence of law enforcement agencies and the criminal justice system leads to the use of scientific practices in criminal investigations.

Principles of forensic science

Forensic science is a profession in which scientific authority points towards the recognition, identification, individualization and evaluation by the employment of all science (physical, natural and law). It implies the utilization of clinical and diagnostic knowledge and skills for the particular requirements of the legal, judicial and police systems. Various specialists are practicing in this field: forensic pathologists, medicolegal consultants, autopsy surgeons, police surgeons, forensic medicine experts, forensic nurses, etc. They have the opportunity to recognize the victims during their initial evaluation. Any loss of evidence can compromise and violate the victim's right to justice. Criminalistics uses scientific methods like finger marks, ballistic trajectory, the study of poisons, investigations on firing and blasting, inquiry of registers and handwriting, microdissection, examining traffic accidents, the study of humans and insects, DNA technology, Automated Fingerprint Identification System and cybercrime to obtain evidence. Forensic science retraces past criminal occurrences through the scrutiny of the physical remnants of that evidence. The results of those analyses and their expert interpretation establish relationships between people, places and objects pertinent to those circumstances. It assembles these results through logical inferences. The following are the seven basic principles of forensic science (Fig. 1.1).

Law of originality
Every artificial or natural object has uniqueness that cannot be matched with any other object e.g. fingerprint

Principle of exchange
Traces are left behind when a crime occurs

Law of progressive change
Changes happen in criminal, the crime scene and objects involved in the crime, thus becoming unidentifiable

Law of differentiation
It emphasizes the need of providing demarcation between sample and specimens

Law of scrutiny
Highlights the need of correct sampling and packaging for use by experts

Law of incidental reality
'Facts do not lie, men can do', i.e. concurrent evidence is as important as an oral one

Law of probability
The findings are made carefully based on all possibilities

Fig. 1.1

Basic principles of forensic science.

Forensic medicine

Forensic medicine is a branch of forensic science where the principles of medical science are applied to help solve legal issues. Forensic medicine deals with crimes against human beings, to furnish equity in the court of law. Forensic casualty requires both health care and legal systems. It is a practice of common sense amalgamated with the implementation of knowledge and experience gained in other branches of medicine.

Definitions

- Forensic medicine is the application of medical knowledge in the administration of justice by correlating such knowledge and applying it to the purpose of the law.
- Forensic medicine can be defined as 'the application of medical and paramedical scientific knowledge to certain branches of law, both civil and criminal.

Classification

- *Clinical forensic medicine:* deals with the inspection of living individuals. (Used in sexual offenses, wound certificate, age estimation)
- *Forensic pathology:* deals with analysis and judgment of autopsy findings in medicolegal investigations.

Importance of forensic science in medical science

- Forensic science deals almost entirely with the crime against persons. Offenses against the human body require the medical opinion to deliver impeccable justice in the court of law.
- Forensic science provides the source of information about medical science to confine the needs of the law. It is mostly an exercise of common sense combined with the application of knowledge and experience acquired in the other branches of medicine.
- The components in forensic science, which are applicable to the medical setting in illustrated in Fig. 1.2. These are observation of facts, interpretation of crime scenes, reconstruction of the events based on a medicolegal examination and the collection of evidence. The scope of forensic science in the medical setting is depicted in Box 1.1.

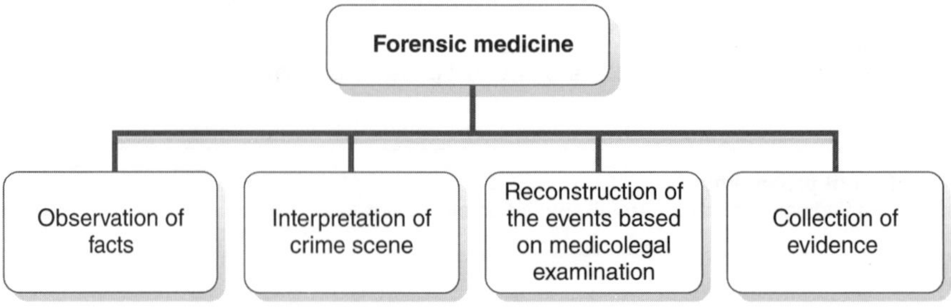

Fig. 1.2

Components of forensic medicine.

BOX 1.1 SCOPE OF FORENSIC SCIENCE IN THE MEDICAL SETTING

1. Screening surviving causality for
   a. Violence-related physical injury
   b. Sexual assault
   c. Child abuse
   d. Domestic violence and battery
   e. Abuse of aged people
   f. Molestation
2. Scrutiny of the assumed criminal
3. Evaluation of self-induced injuries
4. Inquest in road traffic accidents
5. Questioning fitness to drive (alcohol or drug use)
6. Evaluation of psychological health
7. Investigating fitness to be interrogated
8. Documentation of medical findings
9. Interpretation of medical evidence
10. Medicolegal reconstruction of the circumstances and the course of events
11. Presentation of medical evidence in court
12. Medical care of accused in prison and police custody

Forensic nursing

As the practice of medicine becomes more advanced, it becomes mandatory for hospital administrators, physicians and nurses to realize that medical practice can no longer be restricted to curing an ailment. Several cases involve legal problems also. In 1992 the International Forensic Nurses Association (IFNA) was established. A forensic nurse specialist can play a vital role in bridging the gap that exists in attending to the legal sides. It is an area dealing with the scientific role of registered nurses on the medicolegal ground. Its aims are well suited to steer a constructive response to the societal needs of the victims of domestic violence, sexual assault, drug and alcohol addiction, psychological abuse, trauma and other death-related problems. A nursing background along with medicolegal education is suited for this purpose.

Advantages of using the expertise of forensic nurse specialists:

- Helping the physician become free to attend to other medical duties without anxiety
- Collecting and preserving evidence in the emergency department and other situations
- Ensuring proper justice to the victim as evidence is well cared for by a forensically trained nurse
- Assuring significant testimony in court, being the first to see the patient and relatives, and the first to obtain data necessary to consider the reason and pattern of death

If evidence gets destroyed case progression will be affected. So, it is important to recognize the victims and obtain evidence without compromising health care. Health care professionals need to be educated about how to identify forensic victims and preserve the evidence during care.

Forensic science laboratory

Forensic laboratories are facilities where evidence is generated after analysis of physical, chemical, biological or digital examination. A variety of specialists are involved in this and use various disciplines including behavioural forensic science, forensic pathology, forensic anthropology, crime-scene investigation, ballistics, etc.

Forensic laboratories in India

There are four central forensic laboratories in India. The Central Forensic Science Laboratory (CFSL) Hyderabad is a centre of excellence in Chemical Sciences, CFSL Kolkata (the oldest laboratory in India) is distinct in Biological Sciences, CFSL Chandigarh is eminent in Physical Sciences and the fourth laboratory is situated in New Delhi.

The control of all these laboratories is under the Directorate of Forensic Science (DFS) under the Ministry of Home Affairs. Under the supervision of the state forensic laboratory, many forensic laboratories are also present at the regional level in various districts. When evidence is too heavy to transport, or when rapid analysis of evidence becomes imperative, mobile forensic units are dispatched to the crime scene. These units include mini laboratories for on-the-spot analysis, which aids in the further investigation process.

Organization of forensic science laboratory

It is headed by a scientist designated as Director and assisted by scientists at various levels (Deputy Director, Assistant Director, Scientific Officer and other specialists). All the officials of the laboratory, through the Director, investigate the case performances and submit reports to the court.

Various sections in the forensic laboratory

- *Forensic case receipt sector*
  - Case proof that is concealed and the forwarding letter are received here.
  - The specimen is analysed in the concerned laboratory department, and from there the remainder of the samples after testing are sent to this unit to be returned to the police.
  - The reports are handed over at the end.
- *Biological unit*
  - This unit deals with biological evidence (blood, semen, saliva, hair, etc.).
  - The bony parts of the cadaver are examined to determine the species of origin, race, sex, age of the biological material, etc.
- *Serology department*
  - Serological tests are performed here to detect species of origin, blood group substances, enzymes, serum proteins, etc.
  - DNA profiling is also done here.
- *Chemistry division*
  - Chemical analyses of the specimen are carried out here.
- *Toxicology division*
  - Analysis of all materials related to suspected poisoning is ruled out here.
- *Physics division*
  - Analysis of building materials, glass, sand, soil, paint, dirt, etc. is done here.
  - Restoring of erased marks, writings, numbers, etc.
- *Excise and prohibition department*
  - Analysis of liquor, alcohol, blood alcohol level, etc. in the sample is done here.
- *Narcotics unit*
  - Narcotic and psychotropic substances are analysed here.
- *Document examination unit*
  - Paper and ink, handwriting, indentations, obliterations and burned or charred documents are analysed here.
- *Explosives unit*
  - Identification of ballistics, firearms, ammunition, the distance of firing as well as gunpowder residue analysis is done here.
- *Photography unit*
  - Records physical evidence at the crime scene.

- *Fingerprint unit*
  - Processes and examines the evidence for finger marks.
- *Polygraphy*
  - Here lie detectors are used by crime investigators.
- *Voiceprint exploration division*
  - Here it is used to connect a voice to a particular suspect in cases of telephone threats or tape-recorded messages.
- *Other services*
  - Forensic pathobiology
  - Forensic anthropology
  - Forensic entomology
  - Forensic psychiatry
  - Forensic odontology

Violence

Various forms of violence need to be encountered in the practice of forensic nursing. Violence can be domestic violence or public violence. Injuries related to violence are deliberate acts with the intent to cause harm. Domestic violence is a global issue and a major public problem regardless of age, economic status, race, religion, nationality and educational background. Domestic violence has considerable public health consequences as well. It is the responsibility of authorized personnel in the forensic field to coordinate their efforts to uplift their knowledge of domestic violence, collection of evidence and documentation of vital events of physical or sexual violence. In public violence, the victims are more often males. The culprit could be unknown to the victim and of either gender. The place of incident is always a public place. The injuries are declared as inflicted. Violence in the home disturbs women, men and children as victims and the offender could be anyone in the family. The abusive behaviour to dominate in the domestic unit can be any sort of action – physical, sexual, emotional, economic or psychological. These threats of actions or negligence affect another person.

Definition

Violence is an extreme form of aggression that has severe physical harm (e.g. serious injury or death) as its goal (Huesmann & Taylor, 2006).

The United Nations describes violence against women as 'any act of gender-based violence that results in, or is likely to result in, physical, sexual or mental harm or suffering to women, including threats of such acts, coercion or arbitrary deprivation of liberty, whether occurring in public or private life'.

Type of Violence

Depending on the impact of the violence, there are broadly three types of violence.

- Self-directed violence is when violence turned to self such as suicidal acts and self-abusive behaviours.
- Interpersonal violence is the second type of violence that affects a small group of individuals such as intimate partner violence, rape, child abuse and elderly abuse.

- Collective violence is the violence committed by a larger group of individuals such as terrorist acts and mob violence.

Types of violence events

1. *Homicide:* the intentional killing of one person by another
2. *Suicide:* deliberately taking one's own life
3. *Assault:* physical attack by one person upon another
4. *Intimate partner violence:* occurrence of physically violent acts between persons who have an intimate relationship.
5. *Terrorism:* deliberate and planned act of a person or group of people against a civilian population or government for any gain.
6. *War:* a broadscale violence against specific groups of people
7. Workplace violence (WPV): an act of physical, psychological or verbal assault by one worker against another
8. *Child abuse:* injuries intentionally inflicted upon a child, by a parent, caregiver or an adult having the responsibility for the child
9. *Sexual assault:* the act of forcing a person without his or her will to participate in a sexual act

Epidemiology

- All injuries, including those resulting from violent acts, are analysed using three phases of events: pre-event, event and post-event, and three factors: human factor, agent factor and environment factor.
- According to a WHO study, 15%–71% percent of women stated violence (physical or sexual) by their partner; 24%–40% of women reported that their first sexual experience was without consent; 4%–12% of women delineated domestic violence when they were bearing a child.
- Per the WHO South-East Asia Region factuality (2018 statistics), the occurrence of violence against women showed 35% of intimate partner violence. Injuries resulting from violence are responsible for approximately 9% of potential life lost before the age of 75 years.
- According to Global Database on Violence against Women by the United Nations, the prevalence data of violence against women in India is as follows:
  - Lifetime physical and/or sexual intimate partner violence: 28.8%
  - Physical and/or sexual intimate partner violence in the last 12 months: 22%
  - Child marriage: 27.3%
- Per the National Family Health Survey (NFHS) Round 4, the prevalence of intimate partner violence ranges between 3% and 43% in different states of India (Government of India, 2017).
- WPV includes verbal abuse, physical violence, bullying or mobbing, assault and sexual harassment. In meta-analyses on WPV among nurses working in the Southeast Asian region and Western Pacific regions it was found that the pooled prevalence of WPV, verbal abuse, physical violence, threatening behaviour, physical assault, sexual harassment and bullying/mobbing were 58% (CI 51%–64%), 64% (CI 59%–70%), 23% (CI 14%–34%), 30(CI-11%–52%), 21% (CI 8%–38%), 12% (CI 7%–17%) and 25% (17%–33%), respectively. The various determinants of WPV included attributes related to the patient, nurses and organization.

Source of data

Sources of data on violence come from the following:

- Survey research
- Data from clinical settings
- Nongovernmental organizations
- Relevant administrative sources like the National Crime Records Bureau (NCRB) and Census of India

However, actual complete data is still difficult to be captured because of lack of reporting. The magnitude of the problem can be viewed as an iceberg phenomenon. Many sexual violence cases are underreported to the police because women are ashamed or have fear of being blamed.

Sexual abuse – children and women

Sexual abuse has no social, regional, or economic boundaries. It can happen to a person of any gender or age. Women and children are more vulnerable to sexual abuse because of various reasons like considering women and children as harmless victims, gender stereotyping.

- Sexual abuse is any behaviour of a sexual nature that degrades the dignity of a woman.
- Sexual assault includes attacks such as rape or attempted rape, any unwanted sexual contact or threats.

According to the Merriam Webster's Dictionary, *sexual abuse* is the infliction of sexual contact upon a person by forcible compulsion or engaging in sexual contact with a person who is below a specified age or who is incapable of giving consent because of age or mental or physical incapacity.

According to American Psychological Association, *sexual abuse* is unwanted sexual activity, with perpetrators using force, making threats or taking advantage of victims not able to give consent.

Risk factors for sexual abuse

The risk factors of sexual abuse are depicted in Table 1.1, which are broadly classified as individual, community and societal factors. The individual risk factors are young age, alcohol and drug abuse, history of sexual abuse as child, poverty and fear to raise voice. The community and societal factors includes emotionally unsupportive family environment, physical violence and fewer resources in the family, lack of safe employment opportunities, societal norms supportive of gender inequality and tolerance of abuse against women.

Table 1.1 Risk factors for sexual abuse

Individual factors	Community and societal factors
Young age	Emotionally unsupportive family environment
Alcohol and drug use	Physical violence and fewer resources in the family
History of sexual abuse as a child	Lack of safe employment opportunities
Poverty	Societal norms supportive of gender inequality
Fear to raise voice	Tolerance of abuse against women

Consequences/hazards of sexual abuse

- **Exposure to sexually transmitted diseases (STDs):** Violent or forced sex can increase the risk of transmitting many STDs. In forced vaginal penetration, abrasions occur which makes the entry of the virus easily through the vaginal mucosa.
- **Poor mental health:** Sexual violence leads to many psychological and behavioural problems in the victims. Intimate partner violence has a greater impact on the mental health of a person.
- **Unwanted pregnancy:** Unwanted pregnancy is a consequence of sexual abuse. Unintended pregnancy was higher among survivors of sexual violence (54.4%) compared to those who never experienced sexual abuse, as evidenced by a study conducted in South Africa.
- **Increased suicidal tendency:** Females who face sexual harassment are more prone to commit suicide. In Brazil, a study on adolescents showed prior sexual abuse to be a leading factor for suicidal thoughts and attempts.
- **Gynaecological complications:** Forced sex results in various gynaecological complications, which include urinary tract infections, vaginal bleeding, infection, fibroids, irritation in the genital area, chronic pelvic pain.

Approaches for prevention of sexual abuse

The approaches for prevention of sexual abuse is categorized as individual, developmental and community based (Fig. 1.3).

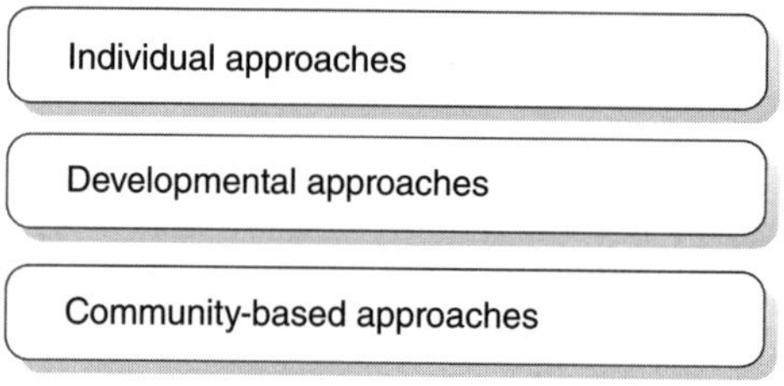

Fig. 1.3
Approaches for prevention of sexual abuse.

Individual approaches

- Care and support by providing economic support for women and families.
- Promoting leadership opportunities for girls. For example, initiatives taken by various governmental and NGOs like Ujjwala, Shakti Shalini and Jagori help to empower women.
- Life skills and other educational programmes: Numerous social/behavioural skills help individuals to adapt and deal efficiently with the challenges of life. These skills include the ability to:
  - think critically, think creatively and solve problems
  - communicate effectively and be confident
  - handle feelings and tension
  - be self-aware

UNICEF states that life skills–dependent attitudes have been successful in educating the younger generation regarding various issues such as drug, alcohol and tobacco use; prevention of pregnancy, HIV/AIDS and other sexually transmitted infections; and promotion of healthy sexuality.

Developmental approaches

- Promote social norms that protect against violence
- Teach gender sensitization and legal awareness

Community-based approaches

- Prevention campaigns include social-emotional learning, instituting and applying workplace policies and solving community-level risks through friendly approaches. Public attitude towards violence can be changed by organizing various awareness programmes and spreading it through media like radio, newspapers.

- School-based programs teach healthy, safe dating and intimate relationship skills to adolescents, along with ensuring safety and monitoring in schools.

Child sexual abuse

Child sexual abuse is the involvement of a child in any form of sexual activity that the child does not fully understand. It may be of any form like fondling, indecent texting through phone or any electronic media, stalking, any form of exhibitionism, showing pornographic content to a child, using the child to make pornographic material, masturbation.

According to WHO, 'Child sexual abuse is the involvement of a child in sexual activity that he or she does not fully comprehend, is unable to give informed consent to, or for which the child is not developmentally prepared and cannot give consent, or that violates the laws or social taboos of society.'

According to the US Centers for Disease Control and Prevention (CDC), child sexual abuse is 'any completed or attempted (noncompleted) sexual act, sexual contact with, or exploitation (i.e. noncontact sexual interaction) of a child by a caregiver'.

Physical and behavioural signs of a sexually abused child

Undergoing sexual abuse in childhood is a traumatic affair. It can have an impact on a person's thinking, actions and feelings enduring a lifetime, leading to physical and psychological health issues. A sexually abused child is likely to exhibit any of the following signs:

Physical signs

- Pain, bruises or evidence of bleeding in the genital area
- Difficulty in walking or sitting
- Blood-stained undergarments
- Recurrent urinary tract infections
- Presence of sexually transmitted disease
- Pregnancy at a younger age

Behavioural signs

- Poor peer relation
- Poor familial relations (with parents, siblings)
- Lack of socialization, playing
- Fearful
- Poor self-esteem
- Avoiding any group activity
- Nightmares
- Bedwetting (inappropriate to the age of the child)
- Thumb sucking
- Sudden change in behaviour
- Poor academic performance
- Substance abuse (in older children)
- Suicidal tendency

Prevention and control of child sexual abuse

The strategies for prevention and control of child abuse include educational awareness, self-defence, support victim and role of government (Fig. 1.4).

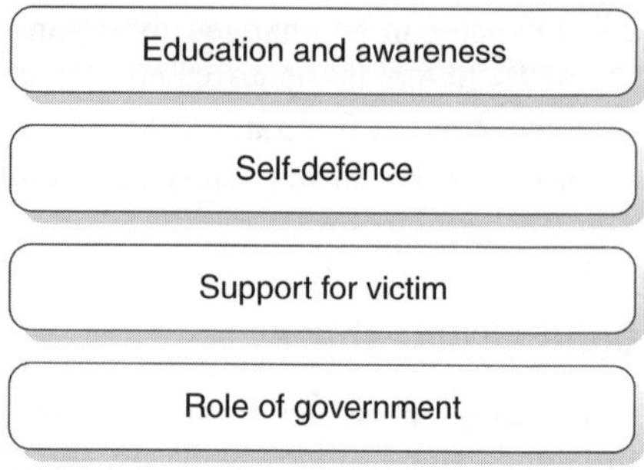

Fig. 1.4

Strategies for prevention and control of child sexual abuse.

Education and awareness

Creating awareness and education acts as primary prevention of child sexual abuse. Parents or caregivers of the child should:

- Speak to the child regarding sexual abuse and the personal and sexual safety.
- Ensure some safety precautions, e.g. if a child is alone, ensure supervision through cameras.
- Ask for details of supervision of child at schools, tuition centres, etc.

To safeguard themselves from perpetrators, children must understand any inappropriate behaviour and should be taught to respond to it.

Inappropriate behaviours of touching include:

- Touching private body parts unnecessarily
- Making a child touch another person's genital area or playing sexual ('pants-down') games

Nontouching behaviours that are inappropriate include:

- Showing porn to a child
- Exhibited a person's genitals to a child
- Demanding children to interact sexually
- Filming a child in sexual poses
- Unveiling a child-to-adult sexual activity through the use of technology
- Sexual gratification by watching a child undress with or without the child's knowledge

Self-defence

Self-defence skills are specifically geared towards minors, acquiring skills for self-protection. These include saying no in perceived situations, avoidance, running off, reporting.

Through self-defence learning competency, they learn to perceive circumstances that put their safety at risk, to avoid similar situations, to protect themselves from danger and to inform a trusted adult immediately afterwards. For long-term effectiveness, it is also important to realize which adults are trustworthy and available for help, in need. These adults could be, for example, school psychologists or teachers in schools.

Support for victim

- Avoid judgment.
- Be with the survivor and stress that you care about his or her well-being and believe his or her statements.
- Be physically present, if the survivor needs medical care or plans to report.
- Offer help and support, if someone thinks of committing suicide.
- Encourage good self-care practices during difficult times.

- Provide helpline numbers for them to contact, e.g. Central Social Welfare Board Police Helpline, 1091/1291, (011) 23317004; Shakti Shalini, 10920.

Role of government

- Policies and laws should be implemented that create gender equality (e.g. equitable access to education, employment and property rights, laws against sexual violence).
- Empowering as well as investing in autonomous women's rights organizations. (In addressing violence against women and policy making.)
- Scaling up survivor-centred services for women affected by violence and their children. It must be comprehensive, accessible and worthy through capacity building of service providers in all sectors (e.g. health, judicial, education, social).
- Through school- and community-based programmes and interventions, challenge norms and attitudes that discriminate against women and girls, especially regarding the acceptability of violence against women,
- Supporting nationalized as well as localized evidence-driven programmes and strategies for prevention.
- End violence against women and girls by promoting community-based and women's organizations.

Legal provisions against violence and sexual abuse

The Government of India has always been proactive in the strengthening of laws and policies to safeguard its citizens from violence and abuse.

- The Immoral Traffic (Prevention) Act, 1956
- The Dowry Prohibition Act, 1961 (No. 28 of 1961) (amended in 1986)
- The Indecent Representation of Women (Prohibition) Act, 1986
- The Commission of Sati (Prevention) Act, 1987 (No. 3 of 1988)
- Protection of Women from Domestic Violence Act, 2005
- The Sexual Harassment of Women at Workplace (PREVENTION, PROHIBITION, and REDRESSAL) Act, 2013
- Protection of Children Against Sexual Offences Bill (POCSO), 2011
- Juvenile Justice (Care and Protection of Children) Act, 2015

Legal aids for help for women in distress

- National Human Rights Commission
- National Commission for Women
- Shakti Shalini
- SAARTHAK
- All India Women's Conference
- JAGORI
- Sakshi – a violence intervention centre
- Saheli – a women's organization
- Nirmal Niketan
- Nari Raksha Samiti
- RAHI (Recovering and Healing from Incest) – a support centre for women survivors of child sexual abuse

Multiple choice questions

1. **The meaning of the Latin word *forensic* is**
   a. public
   b. in open court
   c. of or before the forum
   d. All of the above
2. **Who is considered the father of fingerprint identification?**
   a. Hans Gross
   b. Antisius
   c. Fortunato Fidelis
   d. Francis Galton
3. **Which of the following is NOT a component of forensic medicine?**
   a. Observation of facts
   b. Reconstruction of the events based on medicolegal examination
   c. Punishment to the perpetrator
   d. Collection of evidence
4. **The intentional killing of one person by another is called**
   a. suicide
   b. homicide
   c. assault
   d. intimate partner violence
5. **The Dowry Prohibition Act was enacted in**
   a. 1961
   b. 1962
   c. 1963
   d. 1964

Further Reading

1. Morgan RM. Forensic science. The importance of identity in theory and practice. *Forensic Sci Int Synerg.* 2019;1:239-242.
2. Brettell TA, Butler JM, Saferstein R. Forensic science. *Anal Chem.* 2005;77(12):3839-3860.
3. Houck MM, Siegel JA. *Fundamentals of Forensic Science*. Academic Press; 2009.
4. Saferstein R. *Forensic Science Handbook*. Vol 1. Englewood Cliffs, NJ: Prentice Hall; 2002.
5. Hall AB, Saferstein R. *Forensic Science Handbook*. Vol I. CRC Press; 2020.
6. Byard R, Payne-James J. *Encyclopedia of Forensic and Legal Medicine*. Academic Press; 2015.
7. Peterson C, Florence C, Klevens J. The economic burden of child maltreatment in the United States, 2015. *Child Abuse Negl.* 2018;86:178-183.
8. Leeb RT. *Child Maltreatment Surveillance: Uniform Definitions for Public Health and Recommended Data Elements*. Centers for Disease Control and Prevention, National Center for Injury Prevention and Control; 2008.
9. Mullen P, Walton V, Romans-Clarkson S, Herbison GP. Impact of sexual and physical abuse on women's mental health. *Lancet.* 1988;331(8590):841-845.
10. Choquet M, Darves-Bornoz JM, Ledoux S, Manfredi R, Hassler C. Self-reported health and behavioral problems among adolescent victims of rape in France: results of a cross-sectional survey. *Child Abuse Negl.* 1997;21:823-832.

11. Gomez AM. Sexual violence as a predictor of unintended pregnancy, contraceptive use, and unmet need among female youth in Colombia. *J Women Health (Larchmt)*. 2011;20(9):1349-1356.
12. Bain LE, Zweekhorst MB, de Cock Buning T. Prevalence and determinants of unintended pregnancy in sub-Saharan Africa: a systematic review. *Afr J Reprod Health*. 2020;24(2):187-205.
13. Ameyaw EK, Budu E, Sambah F, et al. Prevalence and determinants of unintended pregnancy in sub-Saharan Africa: a multi-country analysis of demographic and health surveys. *PLoS One*. 2019;14(8):e0220970.
14. Ezegbe HC, Ajayi AI. Association between sexual violence and unintended pregnancy among adolescent girls and young women in South Africa. *BMC Public Health*. 2020;20(1):1370.
15. Barth J, Bermetz L, Heim E, Trelle S, Tonia T. The current prevalence of child sexual abuse worldwide: a systematic review and meta-analysis. *Int J Public Health*. 2013;58(3):469-483.
16. Carson DK, Foster JM, Tripathi N. Child sexual abuse in India: current issues and research. *Psychol Stud*. 2013;58(3):318-325.
17. Belur J, Singh BB. Child sexual abuse and the law in India: a commentary. *Crime Sci*. 2015;4(1):1-6.
18. Srivastava K, Chaudhury S, Bhat PS, Patkar P. Child sexual abuse: the suffering untold. *Ind Psychiatry J*. 2017;26(1):1-3.
19. Abramsky T, Watts CH, Garcia-Moreno C, et al. What factors are associated with recent intimate partner violence? Findings from the WHO multi-country study on women's health and domestic violence. *BMC Public Health*. 2011;11(1):1-7.
20. Hofner MC, Burquier R, Huissoud T, Romain N, Graz B, Mangin P. Characteristics of victims of violence admitted to a specialized medico-legal unit in Switzerland. *J Forensic Leg Med*. 2009;16(5):269-272.
21. World Health Organization. *Guidelines for Medico-Legal Care of Victims of Sexual Violence*. Available at: Whqlibdoc.who.int/publications/2004/924154628x.pdf. Accessed 13 April, 2022.
22. Singh MM, Parsekar SS, Nair SN. An epidemiological overview of child sexual abuse. *J Family Med Prim Care*. 2014;3(4):430.
23. Garg P, Das M, Goyal LD, et al. Trends and correlates of intimate partner violence experienced by ever-married women of India: results from National Family Health Survey round III and IV. *BMC Public Health*. 2021;21:2012.
24. Varghese A, Joseph J, Vijay VR, et al. Prevalence and determinants of workplace violence among nurses in the South-East Asian and Western Pacific Regions: a systematic review and meta-analysis. *J Clin Nurs*. 2022;31(7-8):798-819.
25. Parikh CK. *Parikh's Text Book of Medical Jurisprudence and Toxicology: for Classrooms and Courtrooms*. Medical publications; 1979.
26. Anderson CA, Huesmann LR. *Human Aggression: A Social-Cognitive View*. The Sage handbook of social psychology; 2007:259-287.
27. Huesmann LR, Taylor LD. The role of media violence in violent behavior. *Annu Rev Public Health*. 2006;27:393-415.

UNIT

FORENSIC NURSING

II

Suresh K. Sharma, Nipin Kalal, and Hemlata

Learning objectives

On completion of this chapter, the readers will be able to:

1. Define forensic nursing and expand history and development of forensic nursing.
2. Describe the scope of practice of forensic nurse including setting, areas of practice and its subspecialties.
3. Discuss ethical and legal issues of forensic nursing and role of forensic nurses.
4. Explain Indian Nursing Council and State Nursing Council Acts.

Definition

Virginia A. Lynch, 1986 pioneer of forensic nursing specialty defines forensic nursing as the application of the nursing process to public or legal proceedings, and the application of forensic health care in the scientific investigation of trauma and/or death related to abuse, violence, criminal activity, liability and accidents.

Forensic Health is defined as the application of science to the just resolution of a legal issue (American Academy of Forensic Science, 2010).

History and development

Forensic nursing loomed with the practice of clinical forensic medicine, i.e. as a subspecialty of forensic medicine. Paolus Zacchai, considered the father of forensic medicine, coined the concept to apply medical education to deal with legal questions. Furthermore, he coined the term *clinical forensic medicine* which deals with the principles and practice of clinical medicine to exemplify the questions of judicial proceedings to protect an individual's legal right before death.

Before the inception of forensic nursing, the role of health care professionals was being ignored and in some provinces it was restricted to physicians only. Many other practitioners are involved in this field of forensic medicine, like the medical examiner who is responsible for the investigation of unnatural death.

In the United States, the practitioners of clinical medicine and nursing ignored the forensic issues in the care of living patients. In 1980, US physicians and forensic pathologists recognized the inadequacy of the medicolegal structure and strongly communicated the need for forensic nursing while caring for the living patient. They also stressed that, if vital legal questions were not addressed, the legal issues in healthcare practices may be significantly under-served. In 1983, the first article was published in the *Emergency Medicine Clinics of North America*, where it was revealed that 'medical care of the critically ill patients in the emergency department has caused a significant impact on the practice of forensic medicine'. The same year another article was published titled 'Preserving Evidence in Emergency Department' in the *American Journal of Nursing*. The report highlighted that to safeguard the patient and system, it is very important to conserve and protect the evidence of patients admitted to the emergency department.

In 1988, the US Surgeon General Dr Everett Koop, condemned the response of the social and legal system towards the forensic victim as late. Koop also stated that health care professionals (including doctors, emergency medical technicians, nurses, physician assistants, paramedics and hospital administrators) are responsible to protect the victim's rights and influencing change.

Furthermore, forensic nursing was developed in response to the concerns related to preserving evidence and treatment of a patient suffering from crime-related injuries. Worldwide, the progress of the clinical forensic medicine and forensic nursing was at different pace, with one preceding the other. Clinical forensic medicine was not achieving the same success as forensic nursing.

In 1990, Virginia Lynch developed the integrated practice model for the forensic nursing science as her master's thesis project. In 1991, a year later, following the Lynch's presentation on forensic nursing based on conceptual model, American Academy of Forensic Sciences (AAFS) acknowledged forensic nursing as a forensic specialty. This project was pivotal in the establishment of the forensic nursing as both nursing and forensic specialty. In 1992, forensic nursing pioneers established the International Association of Forensic Nurses (IAFN). The scope was expanded and after 3 years, the American Nurses Association (ANA) granted specialty status to forensic nursing. Furthermore, the fields of medicine, nursing and law worked together for mutual benefits towards the common goal of protecting patients' rights. Later, the resistance was acknowledged from the medical and legal communities.

In spite of the initial resistance, the forensic nursing accelerated the clinical forensic practice in many countries like the United States and Canada. This evolution of forensic nursing science revolutionized the medicolegal management of the forensic patient and reduced the risk of violation of patient legal rights. A brief summary of developmental millstones of forensic nursing is illustrated in Box 2.1.

BOX 2.1 DEVELOPMENT IN FORENSIC NURSING PRACTICE

- 1976: Emergence of Sexual Assault Nurse Examiner (SANE) role in healthcare facilities
- 1991: Formal recognition of Forensic Nursing
- 1992: Foundation of International Association of Forensic Nurses (IAFN)
- 1995: American Nurses Association (ANA) recognized Forensic Nursing as a specialty
- 1997: Published Scope and Standards of Forensic Nursing with IAFN
- 2009: Published the second edition of Scope and Standards of Forensic Nursing
- 2018: Published the revised and updated third edition of Scope and Standards of Forensic Nursing

Integrated Model for Forensic Nursing Science, 1990

The forensic nursing practice model developed by Virgina Lynch (1990) integrates sociology, criminology, clinical and clinical investigation and education. The cyclic nature of this model focuses on continuance, perception and balance. After the identification, verification and demonstration the justice is scaled. This model receives domains from all direction (Fig. 2.1):

- The outer circle frames the components of environment (society, social system and education).
- Centre (internal triangle) reflects legal services, physical, psychosocial, forensic medical and nursing sciences, which is illustrated on justice scale, bundle of public services and the symbol of medicine.

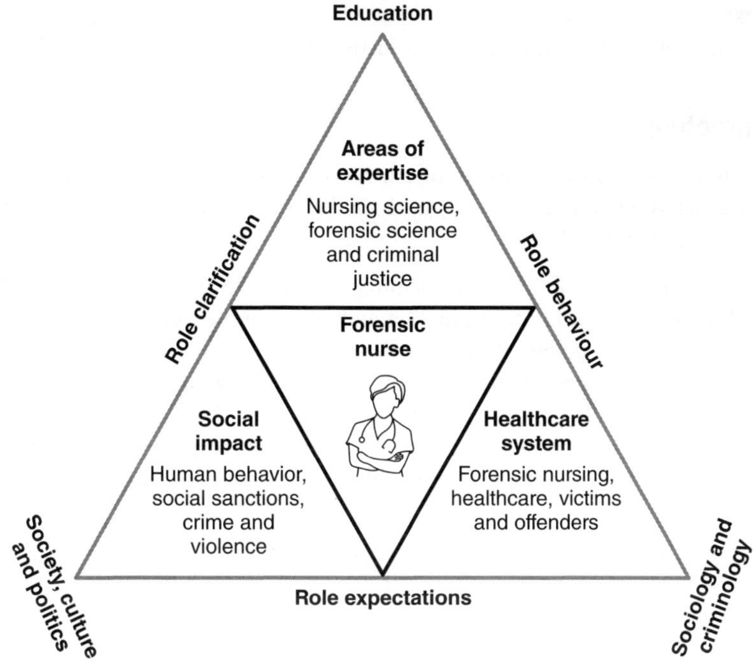

Fig. 2.1

Schematic diagram of a forensic nursing practice model.

- Core: the flame symbolizes the enlightenment of humanity and challenges on expansion of new nursing roles.

Scope

Forensic nursing science combines the concepts and principles of traditional forensic science to investigate and recover the medical evidence. It also provides services to victims, suspects, perpetrators and witnesses of the violence. Scope is the core competency of the forensic cursing. Forensic nurses provide services like Emergency and Trauma services, Prevention of Violence/Elder/Child Abuse or Neglect. Furthermore, forensic nurses preserve and collect the evidence for optimal analysis of the findings.

Setting of practice

Forensic nursing is not limited to a single setting. The application of Forensic Nursing will be broadened as long as any crime, violence and death occurs. The following are the setting of forensic nursing practice:

1. Primary care setting
2. Emergency room department
3. Community or private hospital settings
4. Clinics
5. Legal or investigative arenas

6. Business
7. Educational, industrial and correctional institutes

Area of practice

Forensic Nursing covers the necessity of educational programs for different forensic nursing role. It allows collecting systematic data of physical and behavioural findings with an aim of proving nursing care to patients or victims (Fig. 2.2).

- *Forensic nursing practice:* The forensic nursing process evolves around the individual by providing feedback loop and ensuring re-evaluation and updating the treatment plans. It includes *assessment* of forensic situation, potential victim, *planning* for investigation, *intervention* as documentation about the circumstances, evidence collection, interviewing and provision of care along with appropriate legal agency and *evaluation* of the postinterview care.
- *Violence prevention:* Forensic nursing practice holds the responsibility to convey and communicate violence prevention for promotion of healthier nation and community.

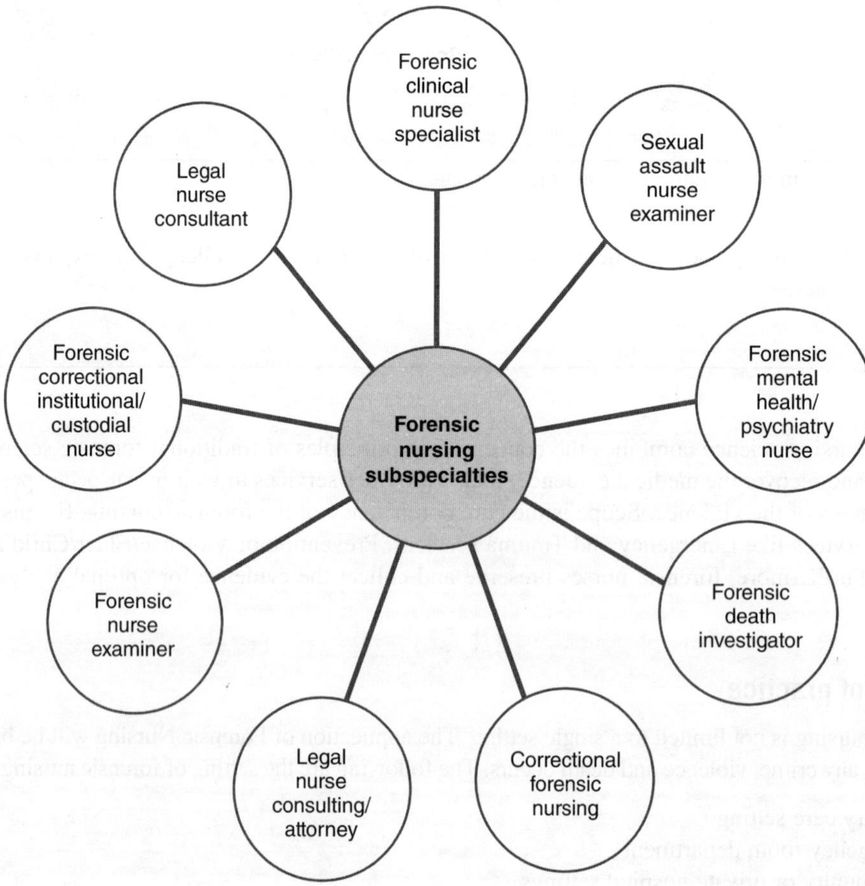

Fig. 2.2

Subspecialties of forensic nursing.

- *Intimate partner violence (IPV):* It is defined as the domestic violence/abuse, gender-based violence including physical, sexual, psychological, spiritual and economic harm by a current or former partner or spouse. In these areas, forensic nurses document the experiences including photographs, collect evidence and perform legal proceedings. They provide supportive nursing care including assessment, intervention and referral of the IPV patient.
- *Mass disaster/community crisis:* Forensic nurses use a biopsychosocial approach to care and preserve the dignity of people suffering from devastation of manmade or natural disaster. They aid the individual to cope with the loss of human life and material resources.
- *Forensic pathology:* They are the first persons to receive the dead bodies, are responsible for police verification and documentation and, also, maintain the mortuary records or any legal formalities related to decedent's presence in the mortuary. They work as mortuary administrator where they are responsible for noting the postpartum staining and rigor mortis prior to artificial cooling and maintain the appropriate temperature of refrigerated storage unit.
- *Forensic traumatology:* In case of trauma, they are specialist to victims where they document the injury with photography, collection of biological fluids, preserve the clothing as an evidence of assault, etc.
- *Forensic toxicology:* Forensic nurses collect the specimens, preserve the appropriate evidence and document the records in a meticulous manner for future presentation.

Roles and responsibilities of a nurse

Forensic nurses are the critical resources for antiviolence efforts. The forensic nursing specialists identify, assess, intervene and evaluate the trauma, disease and death while documenting findings and preserving the evidence for legal functions. The roles and responsibilities of forensic nurse in their subspecialties are elaborated in Table 2.1. A brief summary about the role of forensic nurses is also presented in Box 2.2.

Ethical issues

IAFN stated that ethics are the professional act as a framework for decision-making and dialogue. Ethics are the foundation for the forensic nursing practice. It is very critical to consider the multiple perspectives in creating a foundation for ethical practice as forensic nurses integrate many aspects of nursing science into the practice. There are many ethical issues related to the forensic nursing as they may arise in caring the patient who experience any violence, or did any crime. Table 2.2 illustrates the ethical principles and issues that transpire in forensic nursing practice.

Indian Nursing Council and State Nursing Council Acts

The regulation of nursing education and professional practice of nursing professionals is governed by central law (Indian Nursing [INC] Act) and state law (State Nursing Council [SNC] Act).

Indian Nursing Council Act, 1947

INC is an autonomous body under the Ministry of Health and Family Welfare, Government of India. INC Act, 1947, i.e Act no. 48, was passed by the Parliament of India, which aimed to provide set standards of training for nurses, midwives and health visitors. The prime function of INC is to ensure

Table 2.1 Roles and responsibilities of forensic nursing

Area/subspecialty	Roles and responsibilities
Forensic clinical nurse specialists	They develop and implement the policies related to health care forensic issues and conduct research using elements of forensic nursing science. They evaluate patient outcome while engaging in educating forensic nursing and evidence-based practices. They are qualified with masters or doctoral degree in forensic nursing.
Sexual assault nurse examiners	They provide care to the survivors of sexual assault including rapes. They screen victims for sexual assault as many assaults may go unreported. There is amalgamation of written and verbal questionnaire which help the victim to address assault. They are obliged to protect the patient's legal right while collecting data and evidences required for criminal case. It includes removal of clothing, head to toe examination, collection of specimen for urine, blood and oral swab. They also perform genital examination and STD screening. They are trained in addressing victim's medical, psychological, legal and forensic needs. They are certified as a Sexual Assault Nurse Examiner – Paediatric (SANE-P) or Sexual Assault Nurse Examiner – Adult (SANE-A).
Forensic nurse death investigators (FNDI)	They work within the structure of medical examiner or coroner's department to investigate the death, to support the survivors and family and to explore the impact of death on the community. Also, they perform the investigation of the criminal behaviour in institutionalized care, insurance fraud and in long-term facilities. The certification program of Death Investigator is provided by American Board of Medicolegal Death Investigators.
Legal nurse consultants	They provide declaration to the judicial, criminal justice and health care professionals in case of malpractice, personal injury, product liability and other legal issues related to criminal or civil law. They safeguard the nursing professional in case of any legal issue in the institution. This field is for the registered nurses with a doctorate degree who practice law (civil and criminal) involving healthcare issues.
Forensic nurse examiners	They perform examination through scientific investigation of the scene and circumstances of the death. They also perform investigation of the criminal behaviour in case of abuse, insurance fraud or other aspect of investigative exigency.
Nurse attorney/coroners	Nurse attorneys address legal issues as they intersect with the health care organization.
Nurse coroners	Nurse coroners are state and jurisdictional authorized officer to supply the certification of questioned death, identifying the cause of death and notifying the next of kin.
Forensic correctional, institutional or custodial nurses	They perform medical assessment and give nursing intervention to the patients who are in custody. Their centre of attention is care, treatment and rehabilitation of the persons who are sentenced to jail, prison and juvenile detention centre for violation of criminal status.
Forensic mental health/ psychiatry nurses	They offer therapies to survivors and criminal of violence. They have a master's degree in mental health.
Elder/child/abuse/neglect	They encounter the situation and protect the elder/child from any more trauma. They perform assessment to check and locate for bruises, head injury or sexual abuse. They build trusting relationship to allow the child/ elder to share details of the abuse or neglect. Furthermore, they repost the abuse for legal investigation.

BOX 2.2 ROLE OF FORENSIC NURSE

- Forensic examination
- Collection and preservation the evidence
- Scientific investigation of death
- Identifying elder/child who are at risk of abuse
- Safety of living and deceased victim's body is a priority
- Assisting in development of evidence-based policies and procedure
- Training and continuing education
- Violence prevention

minimum nursing educational standards, recognize nursing qualification and prescribe nursing courses admission criteria and curriculum. INC also grants permissions for establishment of the new school/college and monitor registration and licensing of nurses in SNC and their conduct. The council is composed of elected and nominated members for a tenure of 5 years. They make recommendations to the central government on matters related to nursing education. They conduct inspections of the new institution to recognize the institute for offering different nursing courses. A total 17 sections are illustrated, where each section mentions specific legislative role of council (Box 2.3).

State Nursing Council Act

In year 1948, the State Nurses and Midwives Council (SNC) Act was established under the provision of Nurses and Midwives Act with the aim of 'Better training of Nurses, Midwives and health Visitors'. SNCs are constituted in respective states. It is an autonomous body of the State Government and Department of Health and Family Welfare. The first SNC Act was 'The Tamil Nadu Nurses and Midwives Act, 1926'.

Structure: Respective states regulate the administrative responsibilities and supervise the council of nursing. It consists of the state Governor, Nursing Directorate, State Health Directorate and/or other state organizations.

Table 2.2 Ethical issues related to forensic nursing

Human rights issue	• Protecting patient rights and human dignity • Using/not using physical or chemical restraints • Protection of patient right of research subject • Use of experimental treatments or equipment with patient consent
End-of-life treatment decision	• Treating or not treating against patient/family wishes • Acting against religious practice • Ordering/performing too many procedures • Using or removing life support • Resuscitate or not to resuscitate without knowing the patient's wish • Determining when death occur • Procuring or distributing organs or tissue for transplantation
Patient care issue	• Conflict in nurse–physician or other professional relationships • Neglect in reporting the child/elder abuse • Participating in abortion/fertility treatment against your conscience
Autonomy/informed consent/ confidentiality	• Ignoring patient/family autonomy • Defamation of the duty of keeping confidentiality • Disclosure of the conflict of interest
Commitment to colleagues	• Disclosure/exchange of information regarding the patient • Partnership among forensic nurses and other professional with same interest to eliminate threat to health and justice • Taking credit for others contribution • Disrespect the colleagues and share their ideas with others

BOX 2.3 SECTIONS OF INDIAN NURSING COUNCIL ACT, 1947

1. *Short title, extend and commencement:* This act is named as Indian Nursing Council Act, 1947. It is extended in every state of India, except State of Jammu and Kashmir and it will come into force at once.
2. *Interpretation:* It describes the meaning of words like *Council* as constituted under this Act, *Prescribed* as prescribed by regulations made under Section 16 and *State* register meaning register of nurses in the state.
3. *Constitution and composition of Council:* Council constitute the following members:
   a. One nurse enrolled in state register
   b. Two members elected by head of institutions recognized by the Council
   c. One member each elected by head of institutions in which health visitors are trained
   d. One member each elected by the Medical Council of India (MCI)
   e. One member each elected by the Central Council of the Indian Medical Association (IMA)
   f. One member each elected by the Trained Association of India (TNAI)
   g. Auxiliary nurse-midwives enrolled in state register from four group of states – Group 1: Kerala, Madhya Pradesh, Uttar Pradesh and Haryana; Group 2: Andhra Pradesh, Bihar, Maharashtra and Rajasthan; Group 3: Karnataka, Punjab, Himachal Pradesh and West Bengal; Group 4: Assam, Gujarat, Tamil Naidu and Orissa
   h. The Director General of Health Services (DGHS)
   i. The Chief Principal Matron, Medical Directorate, General Headquarters, ex officio
   j. The Chief Nursing Superintendent, Office of the Director-General of Health Services, ex officio
   k. The Director of Maternity and Child Welfare, Indian Red Cross Society, ex officio
   l. The Chief Administrative Medical Officer (by whatever name called) of each state other than a union territory, ex officio
4. *Incorporation of the Council:* Council constituted under Section 3 shall be a body corporate by the name of the Indian Nursing Council having common seal.
5. *Mode of election:* Elections under Subsection 1 of Section 3 by State Councils shall be conducted in accordance with rules made in this behalf by the respective State Governments, and in case of any dispute decision of the State Government will be considered as final. Elections under that subsection shall be conducted in the prescribed manner and in case of any dispute decision of the Central Government will be considered as final.
6. *Term of office and casual vacancies:* Elected or nominated members, other than a nominated President, will hold office for a term of 5 years. They may resign at any time by writing to the president. Any casual vacancy shall be filled by fresh election or nomination. Members of the Council shall be eligible for re-election.
8. *Officer, committee and servant of Council:* The Secretary of the Council is appointed for 3 years by the Central Government. The Council shall elect from members a Vice-President, an Executive Committee and such other committees for general or special purposes, and also appoint servants as the Council deems necessary to carry out the purposes of this Act.
9. *The executive committee:* nine members, of which seven are from the Council.
10. *Recognition of qualification:* There were two parts of qualification – part 1 schedule shall be recognized qualification and part two is higher qualification.
11. *Effect of recognition:* Any person who holds a recognized qualification will be enrolled in state register and any person with higher qualification will be entered in supplementary qualification in any state register.
12. *Power to require information as to course of study and training and examination:* Every authority of state who grants qualification or higher qualification must furnish time to time information of the Council to meet the Council standards.
13. *Inspections:* Executive Committee appoints the number of inspectors for conduction of inspection and sending the report of the training institutions before any grant or recognition of the institution.
14. *Withdrawal of recognition:* Inspection report is produced to the Council and if any shortfall, the institution is required to send explanation to state government within a certain period. If explanation is not submitted within the time period the Council can withdraw of recognition.
15. *Mode of declaration:* All declarations under Section 10 or Section 14 to *be* published in the Official Gazette. Section A: Maintain the Indian Nurses register in prescribed manner; Section B: Supply 20 copies of State registers after 1st day of April each year.
16. *Power to make regulation:* The Council may make regulations not consistent with this Act; such regulations may provide for property of the Council, elections, meetings, prescribe function of executive committee, power and duties of president and vice president, secretary and other officers, prescribe standard curricula, condition for admission to course of raining, standard of examination and any other matter.

Repeal OF ORDINANCE 13 OF 1947: PART I – Recognized qualifications: General Nursing Certificates (including senior and junior certificates), Diplomas or Degrees in Nursing issued by any of the state councils. PART II – Recognized higher qualifications like Postgraduation in Nursing.

Function: SNC is responsible for conducting the examination for the certificate or diploma nursing courses and register the qualified person as nurse, midwife and auxiliary nurse-midwife or health visitor. SNC maintain the registration of nurses, midwives, health visitors, auxiliary nurse-midwives and *dhais* who have undergone the course of training and passed the examinations and fulfil the condition prescribed in the respective state. Nurse registration board enforces the *Nursing Practice Act.* SNC also provides the NOC (no objection certificates) in case of state to state transfer of the nurses registration to provide licensure to work in other state.

Multiple choice questions

1. **Who is considered as the pioneer of forensic nursing?**
   a. Virginia A. Lynch
   b. Virginia Henderson
   c. Dorothea Orem
   d. Callista Roy
2. **IAFN stands for**
   a. International Alumni of Forensic Nurses
   b. International Association of Federal Nurses
   c. International Association of Forensic Nurses
   d. International Assumption of Forensic Nurses
3. **The outer circle of the Integrated Model for Forensic Nursing Science (1990) encompasses**
   a. society, social system and education
   b. legal services, physical, psychosocial, forensic medical and nursing sciences
   c. enlightenment of humanity
   d. challenge on expansion of new nursing roles
4. **Nurse coroners mainly deals with**
   a. the certification of questioned death
   b. care, treatment of juvenile victims
   c. declaration to the judicial
   d. care to the survivors of sexual assault
5. **Indian Nursing Council Act was enacted in**
   a. 1947
   b. 1946
   c. 1945
   d. 1949

Further Reading

1. Whyte L. Forensic nursing: a review of concepts and definitions. *Nurs Stand.* 1997;11(23):46-47.
2. Forensic Nursing. *Forensic Nurse Death Investigator*. Elkridge, MD: International Association of Forensic Nurses; 2020.
3. Lynch VA Virginia A, Duval JB. *Forensic Nursing Science*. Forensic Nursing. 2011:672. Available at: http://encore.unisa.ac.za/iii/encore/record/C__Rb2386622__SPsychological Assessment in South African context__Orightresult__U__X1__T?lang=eng&suite=cobalt.

4. American Nurses Association and International Association of Forensic Nurses. *Forensic Nursing: Scope and Standards of Practice*. 2nd ed. Silver Spring, MD: American Nurses Association; 2017.
5. Gorea R, Lynch V. Forensic nursing – a boon to the society. *J Punjab Acad Forensic Med Toxicol.* 2003;3(3):32–36.
6. Scannell MJ. "History of forensic nursing," In: *Fast Facts About Forensic Nursing*. Springer publication, 1st edition, 2018:1-10
7. Nurse Key. Evolution of forensic nursing science. In: *Evolution of Forensic Nursing Science*. Available at: https://nursekey.com/1-evolution-of-forensic-nursing-science/.
8. Price B, Maguire K, eds. *Core Curriculum for Forensic Nursing*. Elkridge, MD: International Association of Forensic Nurses; 2016.
9. Valentine JL. Forensic nursing: overview of a growing profession Career Sphere. *Am Nurse Today*. 2018, 13(12):42-44.
10. Duquesne University. *Ethical Practice in Forensic Nursing*. 2019. Available at: https://onlinenursing.duq.edu/blog/ethical-practice-in-forensic-nursing/.
11. Yadav PK. Ethical issues across different fields of forensic science. *Egypt J Forensic Sci*. 2017;7(1):1-10.
12. Ekroos RA. *Exploring Forensic Nursing Ethics and Practice: Roles, Loyalties and Photodocumentation Practices*. PhD Thesis. 2016.
13. Tsunematsu K, Fukumoto Y, Yanai K. Ethical issues encountered by forensic psychiatric nurses in Japan. *J Forensic Nurs*. 2021;17(3):163-172. doi:10.1097/JFN.0000000000000333.
14. Jaivin Jaisingh J, Sridhar KMK. Scope of forensic nursing. *Int J Recent Sci Res*. 2019;10(06):32709-32715. Available at: http://dx.doi.org/10.24327/ijrsr.2019.1006.3528.
15. Hammer R, Moynihan B, Pagliano E. *Forensic Nursing: a Handbook for Practice*. Jones & Bartlett Publishers; 2011:518. Available at: https://books.google.com/books?id=APgVX1WcuYcC&q=forensic+nursing&pg=PP2.
16. Mason T, Lovell A, Coyle D. Forensic psychiatric nursing: skills and competencies: i role dimensions. *J Psychiatr Ment Health Nurs*. 2008;15(2):118-130. Available at: https://www.researchgate.net/publication/5639285.
17. Angela F, Amar LKS. A *Practical Guide to Forensic Nursing: Incorporating Forensic Principles into Nursing Practice*. Sigma Theta Tau International All; 2014:1-406.
18. Bektaş G, Pakiş I. Awareness of forensic cases among nurses. *J Forensic Nurs*. 2021;17(3):1-6.
19. Dash SK, Patel S, Chavali K. Forensic nursing - global scenario and Indian perspective. *J Forensic Leg Med*. 2016;42:88-91. Available at: http://dx.doi.org/10.1016/j.jflm.2016.05.020.
20. Indian Nursing Council. *Indian Nursing Council Act 1947*. Available at: https://indiannursingcouncil.org/uploads/inc-act-1947.pdf.
21. Sharma S. Nursing Practice Act: current scenario and future needs of India. *Nurs J India*. 2017;CVIII(6):250-254.

UNIT

FORENSIC TEAM

III

Jaison Joseph

Learning objectives

On completion of this chapter, the readers will be able to:

1. Identify members of the forensic team and describe the role of the forensic nurse.
2. Outline the comprehensive forensic nursing care of a victim and his or her family.
3. Discuss the key points related to the role of the nurse in forensic evidence preservation.

Forensic team – members and their roles

Forensic health care has become a *multidisciplinary team approach* with an attempt to meet the varied needs of the patients as well as their families. The forensic evaluation involves *holistic assessment* including physical, mental and legal aspects depending on the nature of the problems. The members of the team may vary per the extent of the medical and mental health problems which need to be thoroughly examined through a forensic interview followed by the collection of appropriate evidence. Each member of the team has an integral role in facilitating the best possible outcomes for the beneficiaries (Table 3.1).

Role of nurse in forensic evidence preservation

Forensic nursing is a specialized area of nursing practice that involves the application of nursing principles to handle certain forensic situations such as trauma, domestic violence, sexual assault and drug abuse. The practice settings of the forensic nurse include various health care areas such as hospital emergency settings, private clinics, psychiatric hospital settings and other forensic legal institutions. However, the forensic nurse has to address the holistic care of the patients, such as providing emotional support to the victims, providing care during physical injuries and timely preservation of evidence. Proper and adequate preservation of evidence is a mandated legal document for the victim. Therefore, evidence preservation is an important role in forensic nursing practice.

1. **Observation:** The initial step for evidence preservation is to observe the nature and source of injuries. The nature of trauma might be physical or sexual or emotional which might have resulted from the accident, assault, violence, drug abuse, etc. Head to toe complete assessment of the victim

Table 3.1 Forensic team members and their roles

Team member	Major responsibilities
Forensic medical team	

Forensic medical officer/specialist/forensic physicians/forensic pathologist: MD in forensic medicine after MBBS/ postgraduation degree in forensic medicine	• Conducting forensic medical examination
	• Conducting postmortem examination
	• Issuing certificates such as death certificates and other medicolegal documents
	• Providing expert forensic scientific services such as reporting medicolegal issues to the judiciary system
	• Involvement in teaching and research related to the specialties of forensic medicine
	  ◦ Forensic toxicology: Studying the forensic aspects of alcohol and drugs
	  ◦ Forensic odontology: Studying the forensic aspects of teeth and biting marks
	  ◦ Forensic pathology: Studying forensic aspects of anatomical and functional changes including the blood and body fluids analysis.

Medical practitioners: health care personnel such as general physicians, general surgeons, gynaecologists and those employed in certain settings such as emergency departments	• Assessment and early intervention of the acute physical and emotional needs of the victims • Treatment and referrals for relevant consultation
Forensic nursing team	
Forensic nurse: a registered nurse who has undergone training in forensic nursing.	• Doing a comprehensive evaluation of victims of trauma, domestic violence, sexual assault, drug abuse, and certain death investigation • Conducting forensic interviews including forensic history and documenting forensic evidence • Involvement in the dissemination of education and research related to evidence-based forensic nursing
Forensic clinical nurse specialist: a nurse with a master's or doctoral degree in forensic nursing	• Doing a comprehensive evaluation of patients/victims/dead bodies • Conducting forensic interviews including forensic history and documenting forensic evidence • Involvement in the dissemination of education and research related to evidence-based forensic nursing
Psychiatric forensic nurse: a forensic clinical nurse specialist who has done specialization in mental health/master's or doctoral degree in psychiatric nursing	• Diagnosis and treatment of mental health issues of forensic patients such as sexual assault/rape victims
Forensic nurse examiner/sexual assault nurse examiners (SANE): a trained nurse with the following certifications – sexual assault nurse examiner for adults (SANE-A) or sexual assault nurse examiner for paediatrics (SANE-P).	• Performing accurate head to toe examination and obtaining forensic medical history • Properly collecting and documenting the potential evidence • Ensuring direct nursing care of physical illness for victims of sexual assault • Crisis intervention: assisting the psychological needs of victims of sexual assault

Table 3.1 Forensic team members and their roles—cont'd

Team member	Major responsibilities
Forensic nurse death investigator: a forensic nurse who had undergone a certification program and certified as a death investigator	• Collection of evidence and information related to the manner of death • Assisting in the forensic medicolegal examination of the victim
Miscellaneous forensic team members	
Forensic scientist: having master's degree/doctoral degree in forensic science	• Collecting evidence with credible proofs such as photographs, sketches, fingerprints, body fluids • Analysing the evidence such as drug analysis, DNA analysis, trace evidence analysis • Preparing and accurately communicating the evidence
Forensic psychiatrist: a psychiatrist who has done MD in psychiatry with special training in forensic psychiatry/forensic science	• Assessing and prescribing medications for victims with mental health problems • Providing psychiatric expert advice to the judiciary system such as fitness to stand court trials, admission to mental hospitals
Forensic psychologist: a psychologist with master's degree/doctoral degree in psychology with special training in forensic psychology	• Assessment and psychological treatment of victims with mental health problems • Screening and understanding psychological disorders of criminal defendants • Expert witness and consultant in the field of the criminal justice system
Forensic photographer: with a certified course in forensic science and forensic photography	• Accurately framing and determining the key evidence • Using the appropriate imagining technique to collect photographic evidence

is important to identify the extent of the injury. The collection of the evidence should be undertaken along with observation and physical examination. The vital signs should be properly monitored and the medical need should be met accordingly. The description of the observation should be concise and should provide a clear outlook of general appearance, attitude and behaviour. When proceeding for physical examination, the nurse must ensure that proper informed consent has been taken and it should be conducted in the presence of a nominative representative of the victim to promote safety and comfort.

- *Clothing:* Examination of the clothing is considered critical evidence in forensic studies. Nurses working in the emergency department should attempt to locate and recover the removed clothing especially in case of a suspect of a sexual assault victim. Furthermore, both the fresh and changed clothing should be collected as evidence as the body fluids usually drain into the garments.
- *Skin:* The skin of the victim is a major evidence in medicolegal examination and should be kept unwashed until the collection of evidence is completed. Wearing of proper protective equipment and preservation should be followed during evidence collection to avoid cross-contamination.
- *Bite marks:* These are commonly found in sexual assault and domestic violence such as a child or elderly abuse. The characteristics of the evidence such as location, size, shape, colour and depth

should be properly documented. After the examination and documentation of findings, the area of the bite mark should be properly cleaned initially with a wet swab followed by a dry swab.

The following postmortem changes should be observed by the nurse during forensic observation.

- *Algor Mortis:* This is the cooling of the body after death. The nurse can assess the changes in the body temperature by palpating the body of the deceased.
- *Livor mortis:* This is the purplish-red discoloration of the body after death due to the pooling of blood in the vascular system. The nurse can observe this thorough inspection of the area of discoloration which can be most noted in the gravity-dependent areas.
- *Rigor mortis:* This is the stiffening of the body due to biochemical changes of muscles after death. It can be assessed through both inspection and palpation.
- *Drying of tissues:* The discoloration of the mucus membrane, sclera, lips and genitals can be easily observed in a deceased patient through inspection.

2. **Recognition:** The materials that can be seen with the naked eye can be easily identified packaged accordingly. However, some of the trace evidence need not be detected on general visual examination that needs to be supported with illumination techniques such as magnification, using high-intensity lighting, lasers. Moreover, evidence needs to be recognized based on certain characteristics.
   - *Nature of injury:* Depending on the type of trauma, special attention must be given to tracing the materials. For example, in case of blunt or sharp trauma, the selected evidence needs to be identified, such as the number of bullet holes and bloodstains in clothing. Similarly, depending on the poison ingested, the articles should be preserved. For example, in case of suspected food poisoning, the search for gastric contents and blood must be initiated.
   - *Time:* Timely identifying the evidence is of prime importance in forensic nursing. For example, saliva should be identified early within 48 hours for better preservation of DNA analysis. In case of sexual assault, the forensic exam can be initiated within 96 hours for accurate estimation of trace evidence. However, bite marks and other injuries can be traced within 5 days of the attack.
3. **Collection of evidence:** The collection of evidence is an important step in the evidence preparation because it links the situations of the victims to be investigated. While collecting, the nurse needs to follow certain forensic principles such as adherence to sterile technique to prevent contamination and preservation of the accuracy of findings. The nurse should be competent enough to collect all the minute materials or trace evidence that might influence the forensic findings. Some forensic techniques for the collection of evidence are as follows:
   - *Cutting:* This is the separation of an item containing the evidence by using a clean cutting device.
   - *Combing:* The clear evidence materials from the hairs can be removed by using a clean comb or a brush.
   - *Picking:* The separation of the evidence using some picking materials such as forceps is an important technique in evidence collection. The sample should be promptly kept in a separate envelope or box to avoid loss or contamination.
   - *Tape lifting:* Some evidence such as hair and fibre materials need to be removed with the aid of adhesive tapes to protect from contamination and better comparison.
   - *Vacuum sweeping:* This is the removal of the suspected evidence with the aid of a vacuum cleaner. This technique has a demerit of the collection of a large number of extra materials apart from the desired samples resulting in cross-contamination.
   - *Scrapping:* A clean spatula is used to remove the trace evidence such as under the fingernails.
   - *Clipping:* Evidence from the fingernails can be collected using clean scissors or clippers.

4. **Preservation:** Depending on the nature of the evidence, the materials should be appropriately preserved. There are certain principles for packaging and preserving forensic evidence.
   - All the relevant items must be preserved in sealed envelopes/boxes/containers, per the type of samples. For example, small and very minute samples should be kept in clean unused primary containers.
   - Appropriate labelling must be done, e.g. label as 'storage under room temperature' or 'storage under frozen temperature'.
   - Packages should not be mixed and be stored separately.
   - Biological evidence should be air-dried before packaging and preserved in a cool and sterile environment.
5. **Documentation:** Before documentation of findings, the nurse must obtain consent to document. There are three components in forensic documentation – written component, diagrammatic component and photographic component. The written component must be clear, legible and accurate. The forensic nurse uses objective observation throughout the documentation procedure. Diagrammatic component includes the detailed description of evidence with the aid of relevant diagrams. Photographic component is the most accurate and representative of the evidence. Ensure that photographs are arranged per the sequence such as begin with a full-body photograph followed by a close-up. Furthermore, be sure that the photographs are adequately labelled indicating the name of the patient, date and time of photography with the name of the photographer. The following descriptions of evidence should be documented:
   - The location, size, shape, colour and depth of injury
   - Type and size of the traced materials
   - Unusual marking and stains, if any

   Avoid common errors in documentation such as the use of jargon and vague statements.
6. **Forwarding biological samples for forensic examination:** A clear, well-documented chain of custody tracking record should be maintained with a clear description of items, time and date of collection, and packaging with appropriate seal and signature. This is called a chain of custody record.

Comprehensive forensic nursing care of victim and family

Forensic nursing is a new and evolving discipline in the nursing profession. Being the largest number among health care personnel, the nurses are an important resource to the application of forensic science in health care. Nurses employed in the emergency hospital care setting, already possess certain skills related to forensic science such as evidence collection and preservation. However, nurses must possess certain additional skills to deliver comprehensive and holistic care to be recognized as forensic nurses. These fundamental skills include forensic interviewing and examination skills, evidence preservation skills, forensic documentation skills and the knowledge of forensic care per the type of victims. The following are the various aspects of care a nurse has to be performed within the realms of forensic nursing:

- **Physical aspects:** The essential care for a forensic nurse is to provide the need-based physical care of the victim.
  a. ***Custodial emergency care:*** Depending on the type of injury or illness, the nurse has to support with prompt nursing care such as assessment of vital signs and assuring interventions as ordered.

b. ***Conduct or assist during forensic examination:*** As the primary care provider, the nurse has a pivotal role in the forensic examination of the victims. The following principles have to be followed while conducting or assisting during forensic examination:
   - Obtaining written informed consent from the victim or nominated representative for the procedure.
   - Accurately recording the history of the incident including types of violence or injury, per the area of involvement.
   - Head to toe assessment with special focus on the trace evidence such as fingernail scrapings, presence of a foreign body inside the body orifices, areas of tenderness.
   - Assessment and collection for certain body fluids such as seminal fluid in case of sexual assault, saliva, and blood in case of drug abuse

- **Psychosocial aspects:** The psychosocial care of the victim is an essential role of the forensic nurse to meet the emotional and social needs. The acronym 'LIVES' is a counselling strategy to meet the immediate emotional needs of the victim:
  a. ***Listen:*** The nurse should actively listen to the victim empathetically and understand the concerns without any predetermined judgments.
  b. ***Inquire:*** The nurses working with victims should initially inquire about the various emotional needs and social concerns.
  c. ***Validate:*** After inquiring about various needs, the nurse should help the victim to accept reality without blaming himself or herself or others. This can be conveyed by saying, 'It is not your fault; you are not supposed to blame yourself.'
  d. ***Enhance safety:*** The nurse should explore and discuss the possible plans and options to prevent and protect the victim from similar experiences. The nurse should discuss the probable safety plans and the avoidance of risky situations.
  e. ***Support:*** The nurse should assess the individual coping mechanism of the victim and further ensure and enable the victim to use the existing social support.
- **Cultural and spiritual aspects:** The forensic nurse has a role to provide culturally and spiritually congruent care for the victim. The goal of forensic nursing is to promote the positive integration of personality by fostering preexisting cultural and spiritual beliefs.
  a. Understand the cultural identity of the individual by exploring the cultural practices and beliefs of the victim before conveying caring and optimism.
  b. Assess the cultural norms and culturally normative behaviours.
  c. Explore the unique or unusual symptoms of the victim based on the cultural adaptation and entity.
  d. Assess the individual perception of the victim and validate the cultural explanation of illness.
  e. Respect the personal belief of the victim according to his or her culture and spirituality.
  f. Establish a verbal contract and enable survival skills based on spiritual strength.
  g. Offer peace of mind by fostering spirituality.
  h. Ensure a culture-specific forensic interview. This can be achieved by granting to follow certain rituals during the therapeutic process such as prayer, allowing to fix the date of interview sessions according to religious beliefs.
  i. Maintain a culturally relevant nurse–patient relationship.
- **Legal aspects:** The forensic nurse has the role of an advocate and should be a resourceful person for the victim. The forensic nurse should be diligent enough to protect the rights and understand the victims as a whole.
  a. Assess the intention and ability of the perpetrator (the person who committed the harmful act).
  b. Do comprehensive mental status examination of the victim.

c. Assess the ability of the victim to carry out the court trails.
d. Act a resource person to ensure the available legal support.
e. Perform and prepare accurate documentation of the examination.
f. Support the victim's self-understanding and convey an attitude of openness towards the his or her explanations before arriving at any forensic conclusion.

- **Assist forensic team in care beyond the scope of their practice:** As nurses are working throughout the health care system, they have a role to assist the forensic team beyond the scope of their practice. The baseline knowledge of the nurse in the health care delivery system can help the nurse to enhance competent care and further minimize the negative consequences to the victim.
  a. Apart from providing emotional and acute medical care, further assist the team with accurate evidence preservation.
  b. Collaborate with a multidisciplinary team depending on forensic investigations and therapeutic procedures.
  c. Be involved in research activities to develop guidelines for forensic examination and evidence preservation, per the areas of health care.
  d. Conduct quality improvement programs to familiarize with the concepts and skills of forensic nursing and roles including legal proceedings.
- **Admission and discharge/referral/death of the victim of violence:** The forensic nurse has an extended role during admission and discharge of the victim and death of the victim of violence.
  a. Collect a proper history regarding the circumstances surrounding the incident including the death of the victim after admission to the health care setup.
  b. Appropriately collect the available biological and physical evidence during the admission period.
  c. Generally, forensic cases are admitted through the court system. Therefore, ensure the presence of a legal representative such as police personnel during forensic admission.
  d. Every nursing care during the stay should be directed based on the admission order of the concerned medical practitioner. Furthermore, every effort must be taken to avoid absconding of the victim during the hospital admission period.
  e. Maintain accurate information of the victim during the hospital stay including their belongings. This includes the name and details of visitors, unusual or naturalistic behaviour of the victim.
  f. Ensure the discharge of the victim after obtaining the discharge summary from the concerned authority.
  g. Affirm that all the belongings and personal inventories are handed over to the victim during the discharge procedure.
  h. The death of the victim of violence must be certified by the concerned doctor in charge. It should be timely intimated and delivered to the concerned legal representative such as family members, police personnel.
  i. Ensure that the dead body is packed per the available protocol of the respective institution.
- **Responsibilities of the nurse as a witness:** Depending on the forensic issues, nurses may have to assume the role of a witness in some forensic cases. The nurse must prepare himself or herself to accurately represent and express the evidence during legal proceedings.
  a. Before appearing as a witness in the court, read all the relevant documents and ensure that the documentation is performed per the principles of forensic science.
  b. Testify himself or herself with rehearsal to uphold professional dignity and accountability.
  c. Actively listen to the questions and in case of clarifications request to repeat the same.
  d. Maintain proper eye-to-eye contact and state the fact as it is.

e. In case of any objection, stop arguments and wait for the judge's decision.
f. Avoid manipulation of evidence and state the facts per the observation and preservation of findings.

Multiple choice questions

1. Study of the forensic aspects of anatomical and functional changes including the blood and body fluids analysis is called
   a. forensic toxicology
   b. forensic odontology
   c. forensic pathology
   d. forensic psychiatry
2. The initial step for evidence preservation in forensic medical examination is called
   a. observation
   b. recognition
   c. collection
   d. preservation
3. The purplish-red discoloration of the body after death due to the pooling of blood in the vascular system is called
   a. livor mortis
   b. algor mortis
   c. rigor mortis
   d. drying of tissues
4. Which of the following is/are the forensic technique(s) for the collection of evidence?
   a. Cutting
   b. Combing
   c. Clipping
   d. All of the above
5. The person who committed the harmful act is called
   a. victim
   b. perpetrator
   c. delinquent
   d. scapegoat

Further Reading

1. Lynch VA. Forensic nursing: diversity in education and practice. *J Psychosoc Nurs Ment Health Serv.* 1993;31(11):7-9.
2. Lynch MJ. The autopsy: legal and ethical principles. *Pathology.* 2002;34(1):67-70.
3. Lynch VA. *Clinical forensic nursing: A descriptive study in role development.* The University of Texas at Arlington; 1990.
4. Lynch VA, Duval JB. *Forensic Nursing Science.* Amsterdam: Elsevier Health Sciences; 2010.
5. Lynch VA. Forensic nursing science: global strategies in health and justice. *Egypt J Forensic Sci.* 2011;1(2):69-76.
6. Gorea RK, Lynch VA. Forensic nursing–A boon to the society. *J Punjab Acad Forensic Med Toxicol.* 2003;3(3):32-36.

7. Amar A, Sekula LK. *A practical guide to forensic nursing: incorporating forensic principles into nursing practice*. USA: Sigma Theta Tau; 2015.
8. Trujillo AC, Delapp TD, Hendrix TJ. A practical guide to prevention for forensic nursing. *J Forensic Nurs*. 2014;10(1):20-26; quiz E1-2.
9. Sekula LK, Burgess AW. Forensic and Legal Nursing. In Wecht CH, Rago JT. *Forensic Science and Law* 2005 Dec 22 (pp. 629-656). Florida: CRC Press..
10. Gorea RK, Jasuja OP, Lynch V, Singh KA. Forensic nursing in India-need of the hour. *J Punjab Acad Forensic Med Toxicol*. 2002;2:49.
11. Campbell JC. Nursing assessment for risk of homicide with battered women. *ANS Adv Nurs Sci*. 1986;8:36.s1.
12. Ferrell JJ. Forensic aspects of emergency nursing. *Emerg Nurse Core Curriculum*. 2007;6:1025-1032.
13. Hammer RM, Moynihan B, Pagliaro EM, eds. *Forensic Nursing: A Handbook for Practice*. USA: Jones & Bartlett Publishers; 2011.
14. Langness M, Zweig JM, Tiry E, Henderson E, Stahlmann N, Bastomski S. Examining the Implementation of the National Protocol for Sexual Assault Medical Forensic Examinations. *J Forensic Nurs*. 2022 Apr-Jun 01;18(2):67-77.
15. Asci O, Hazar G, Sercan I. The approach of prehospital health care personnel working at emergency stations towards forensic cases. *Turk J Emerg Med*. 2015;15(3):131-135.
16. Scannell MJ. *Fast facts about forensic nursing: what you need to know*. New York: Springer Publishing Company; 2018.
17. World Health Organization. *Health Care for Women Subjected to Intimate Partner Violence or Sexual Violence: A Clinical Handbook*. Geneva: World Health Organization; 2014
18. World Health Organization. *Strengthening Health Systems to Respond to Women Subjected to Intimate Partner Violence or Sexual Violence: A Manual for Health Managers*. Geneva: World Health Organization; 2017.
19. Filmalter CJ, Heyns T, Ferreira R. Forensic patients in the emergency department: Who are the and how should we care for them? *Int Emerg Nurs*. 2018;40:33-36.
20. Meera T, Singh KP. Forensic nursing: an evolving specialty. *J Med Soc*. 2017;31:141-142.

UNIT

INTRODUCTION TO THE INDIAN CONSTITUTION

IV

Sonali Banerjee

Learning objectives

On completion of this chapter, the readers will be able to:

1. Describe the Indian Constitution.
2. Explain about fundamental rights of an individual.
3. Discuss about the salient features and implications of fundamental rights.
4. Enlist the fundamental rights.
5. Explicate in depth about the rights of the accused.
6. Elucidate in detail about the rights of the victim.

The Indian Constitution

The ultimate law of any nation is its constitution, which delivers the legal outline aimed at the government. It also entitles the authorities and duties of the branches or agencies of the government. Furthermore, it liaisons the connection between the government and its people. Elementary rights and responsibilities are pronounced for the citizens, and generally it creates the root for the voting system in India.

A constitution is the ultimate law which provides the framework of the government, prime functions of various structures of the government and the principles on which the structure of the government shall function. Under the provision of Cabinet Mission Plan, in 1946, foundation of the Constituent Assembly was done with the objective to draft the Indian Constitution. The Assembly had societal representation, even though it was not formed by direct election by people, as it was partially nominated and partially elected. Indian Independence Act was passed in 1947, which gave complete authority to the Constituent Assembly to frame the constitution. The assembly comprised eminent leaders like Jawaharlal Nehru, Dr Rajendra Prasad, G.B. Pant, Abdul Ghaffar Khan, Sardar Patel and Maulana Azad, under the mentorship of Chairman Dr B.R. Ambedkar. The preliminary meeting of assembly was held on 9 December 1946. The constitution was drafted and published in January 1948. Subsequently it was put forth for public opinion before finalizing. The constitution of India was adopted by the constituent assembly on 26 November 1949 and the President Dr Rajendra Prasad signed it. The Constitution of India finally came into force on 26 January 1950.

INDIAN CONSTITUTION AND ITS SALIENT FEATURES

- **Written constitution.**
- **Lengthiest constitution** with 25 parts and 12 schedules. Each part contains several articles, so 395 articles in totality.
- **Dual feature**: rigid as well as flexible.
- **A parliamentary government**:
  - The constitutional head of the state is the Indian President.
  - The head of the Council of Ministers having real executive power is vested on the Prime Minister.
- **Single citizenship**
- **Federal and unitary** constitution.
- **Six fundamental rights are** assured to the citizen of India.
- **Eleven fundamental duties** are assigned to the Indian citizens.
- Each citizen above the age of 18 years has **right to vote.**
- Recognized as **secular state.**
- **Integrated independent and impartial judiciary**.
- Combination of **parliamentary sovereignty and judicial supremacy.**
- Government has **three-tier system.**
- **Includes independent bodies** like Election Commission, State Public Service Commission, Union Public Service Commission
- **Provision for emergency situations** like national emergency, state emergency and financial emergency

The Fundamental Rights

These are the rights of the Indian citizens and are deliberated in the third part, also known as Magna Carta of the Indian Constitution. Equivalence in every facet is granted by fundamental rights; this is regardless of race, colour, caste, religion, birthplace or gender. Articles 12–35 of the Indian Constitution detail about such fundamental rights of the citizen.

Protection of the rights and liberties of Indian citizen against the powers entrusted to the government are aimed by fundamental rights, which eventually means that these rights limit the supremacy of government. No law can be made by the government which forbid the rights of the citizens. However, these rights are not imperative to be followed and can be adjourned during circumstances which pose as an emergency across the country (discussed later in the chapter). Some of the rights like right to movement were suspended amidst the COVID-19 pandemic, when the entire nation followed lockdown norms (Moore SA et al., 2020). All these rights are available against the arbitrary action of the state.

Fundamental rights are known with the name because of two reasons:

- Rights are protected by the constitution.
- Rights are justiciable, i.e. if they are violated then the individual can appeal to the court of law.

Previously there were seven fundamental rights in the Constitution. Right to property has been now considered as only a legal right after the 44th Constitutional amendment in 1978. Hence, presently there are only six fundamental rights. It is now only a legal right. All the facets related to fundamental rights are discussed gradually in this chapter (Table 4.1). The salient features of fundamental rights are illustrated in Fig. 4.1.

Table 4.1 Brief description of Fundamental Rights

Fundamental rights	Article number	Description
Right to equality Articles: 14–18	*14*	Equality before law
	15	Prohibition of discrimination on grounds of religion, race, cost, sex or place of birth
	16	Equality of opportunity in matters of public employment
	17	Abolition of untouchability
	18	Abolition of all titles except military and academic
Right to freedom Articles: 19–22	*19*	Protection of six rights concerning the freedom of: Speech and expression Assembly Association Movement Residence Profession
	20	Protection with respect to conviction for offences
	21	Right to life and personal liberty
	21 A	Right to elementary education
	22	Protection against arrest and detention in certain cases
Right against exploitation Articles: 23–24	*23*	Prohibition of traffic in human beings and forced labour
	24	Prohibition of employment of children in factories, etc.
Right to freedom of religion Articles: 25–28	*25*	Freedom of conscience and free profession, practice and propagation of religion
	26	Freedom to manage religious affairs
	27	Freedom as to payment of taxes for promotion of any particular religion
	28	Freedom as to attendance at religious instruction or religious worship in certain educational institutions
Cultural and educational rights Articles: 29–30	*29*	Protection of interests of minorities
	30	Right of minorities to establish and administer educational institutions
Right to constitutional remedies Articles: 32–35	*32*	Habeas corpus Certiorari Prohibition Mandamus Quo warranto
	33	Power of Parliament to amend the rights deliberated by this part in their application to forces, etc.
	34	Restriction on rights conferred by this part while martial law is in force in any area
	35	The authority to make laws, to give effect to certain specified fundamental rights shall vest only in the Parliament and not in the state legislatures

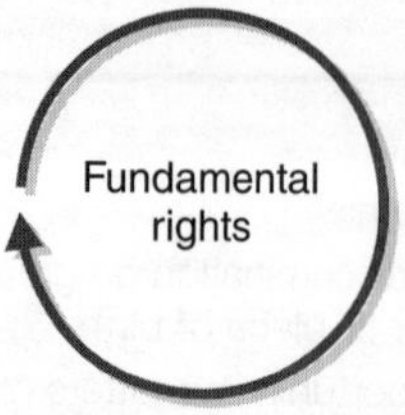

- Granted to citizens of India
- Justiciable
- Amendable
- Safeguarded and defended by the Supreme Court
- Suspended during national emergency
- Parliament restricts the application to special services
- Limits the state authority
- Confers privileges to the citizens

Fig. 4.1

Salient features of fundamental rights.

IMPLICATION OF FUNDAMENTAL RIGHTS

- Provide foundation to democratic India.
- Keeps a check on the governmental powers.
- Societal equality and justice are ensured.
- Confirms liberty, dignity and respect of the citizens of India.
- Ensures the protection of minorities and weaker section of the society.
- Rights facilitate the essential circumstances for protection of Indian citizens.
- Safeguards rule of law in India.

Fundamental Rights and their suspension

- At the time of national emergency as mentioned under article 352, fundamental rights of the citizens can be deferred.
- National emergency may be in the form of external aggression or war attack.
- Article 358 states that the six fundamental rights, as subset of Article 19, are immediately/ inevitably suspended once there is a declaration of national emergency.
- Article 359 has the clause for suspension of other rights. In such case, the President of India issues a discrete notification.
- Whereas rights cited under Articles 20 and 21 cannot be suspended under any circumstances.
- Fundamental rights remain unaffected by Constitutional emergency and financial emergency.

Rights of the accused

The second half of this chapter deals in detail about the two following topics:

- Rights of the accused
- Rights of the victim

An accused cannot be compared with or treated same as a convicted individual. Anyone accused has a right to be considered innocent until the charge is proven; this is affirmed by the Bill of Rights Ordinance, 1991. The Indian Constitution grants certain fundamental rights to the accused individuals (Table 4.2). These rights are allowed before, during and after the progression of any enquiry or any offence related trial for which the individual is accused. These rights support the accused to be protected whilst counter with unlawful or arbitrary arrest.

Table 4.2 Rights of the accused

Article	Description
Article 14 **Right to equality**	This fundamental right confirms that an innocent citizen should never be punished under law and thus facilitates a fair representation in the criminal procedure.
Article 20 **Protection in respect of conviction for offences**	**(1)** No person shall be convicted of any offence except for violation of a law in force at the time of the commission of the Act charged as an offence, nor be subjected to a penalty greater than that which might have been inflicted under the law in force at the time of the commission of the offence. **(2)** No person shall be prosecuted and punished for the same offence more than once. **(3)** No person accused of any offence shall be compelled to be a witness against himself.
Article 22 **Protection against arrest and detention in certain cases**	**(1)** No person who is arrested shall be detained in custody without being informed, as soon as may be, of the grounds for such arrest nor shall he be denied the right to consult, and to be defended by, a legal practitioner of his choice. **(2)** Every person who is arrested and detained in custody shall be produced before the nearest magistrate within a period of 24 hours of such arrest excluding the time necessary for the journey from the place of arrest to the court of the magistrate and no such person shall be detained in custody beyond the said period without the authority of a magistrate. **(3)** No law providing for preventive detention shall authorize the detention of any person for a period longer than 3 months unless • an advisory board consisting of persons who are qualified to be appointed, such as judges of high court, have reported before the expiration of the said period that there is in its opinion sufficient cause for such detention. • nothing in this clause shall authorize such detention beyond the period specified by any law made by Parliament **(4)** When any person is detained in pursuance of an order made under any law providing for preventive detention, the authority making the order shall, as soon as may be, communicate to such person the grounds on which the order has been made and shall afford him the earliest opportunity of making a representation against the order.

Under Constitutional Law

Apart from above-discussed Constitutional laws, there are rights of the accused as decided by the Criminal Laws. Criminal Procedure Code (CrPC) or the Code of Criminal Procedure was passed in 1973 and came into action from 1 April 1974. This Code is the key law-making administrative procedure of functional criminal law in India. Such laws are discussed below.

Pretrial rights of accused in India

These rights facilitate a convicted individual with noninterference in the independence and liberty. The pretrial stage is the first stage of any trial. The police officials can arrest an accused and search all property and belongings on the basis of a filed FIR. The period preceding to the start of a court trial is tremendously critical. So, the following rights are ensured to an accused:

- *Presumption of innocence:*
  - The essence of criminal trial lies in that the accused is to be presumed innocent until a charge is verified against the accused without any reasonable doubt. It is always ensured that not a single innocent should suffer or be punished, even if 10 guilty persons are set free.
- *Right to information/to know the grounds of arrest:*
  - When an individual is arrested without warrant, the person has the right to know the full particulars of offence for which he or she is being arrested.

    (Section 50(1) of CrPC)
  - Furthermore, if the person is arrested with warrant, he or she must be notified the particulars of such warrant, or even show such warrant if desired.

    (Section 75 of CrPC)
- *Right to have bail:*
  - The right of accused individuals consents them to file a bail request to be free from jail custody.
  - Indian law facilitates three specific types of bail:
    - Anticipatory bail
    - Interim bail
    - Bail by a bond
  - Only bailable offence can be allowed for application of bail.
  - However, prior to an arrest, a person with the help of a criminal lawyer can also plea for an anticipatory bail.
  - Any individual, accused of a bailable offence but arrested without a warrant, should be informed by the law enforcers that the individual is eligible to be freed on bail after payment of a warranty.
- *Right to be presented before a magistrate without delay:*
  - The legal authority/police have to present the individual before the Judicial Officer/Magistrate within 1 day per the CrPC Sections 56 and 76. The accused is brought to the Magistrate regardless that the arrest was done with or without a warrant.
- *Right against wrongful arrest:*
  - In India, an accused is facilitated with the rights only in circumstances of issue of legal document like a warrant. The person must be presented in front a Judicial Magistrate within a day of the arrest. This is clearly mentioned in Section 57 of CrPC and Article 22(2) of Constitution.
- *Right to accused of privacy and protection against unlawful searches:*
  - With a meagre speculation of an offence, the privacy of the individual accused of crime cannot be violated by the law enforcement agency.
  - In India, legal authorities do not have the right to pursuit the property of an accused in absence of a search warrant.
- *Right to free, fair and speedy trial:*
  - Just and impartial justice is given to the accused person as early as possible. Trial should be conducted so as to avoid the concept of 'justice delayed is justice denied'.
  - Along with this, the accused must have enough time to prepare a defence.
  - Sometimes the location (venue) of a trial is shifted for good cause, such as security or potential influence of public sentiment.

- *Right to consult a legal practitioner/lawyer/counsel:*
  - For criminal offence, an experienced lawyer can be approached by the accused so as to seek professional help as his or her right. Fundamental rights, i.e. Article 22(1) of the Constitution of India, protects the accused by facilitating with a lawyer and it cannot be denied in any circumstance. This is further reinforced by CrPC Section 50(3), which specifies that the accused has the right to be defended by an advocate of preference against whom proceedings are started.
- *Right of free legal aid:*
  - An accused citizen has the right to hire an attorney of the court to defend him/her.
  - Furthermore, the State facilitates a free of cost legal aid to the accused for court representation in circumstances when he or she cannot financially bear the expenses of a lawyer.
  - The accused has the right to receive free legal aid and this is the responsibility of the magistrate and court to notify the accused.
- *Right against self-incrimination:*
  - Per the Indian Constitution Article 20(3), an accused cannot be compelled to be a witness against himself or herself.
  - The accused is protected from being enforced to disclose incriminating evidences by the abovementioned right. It also averts the practice of torture or other means to force revelations from the accused.
- *Right against double jeopardy:*
  - Article 20(2) of the Constitution enforces that trial or punishment cannot be done more than one time to an individual for the same crime.
- *Right against the ex post facto law:*
  - An Indian citizen cannot be tried for an act which was earlier considered a crime but presently it is considered a noncriminal. This implies that the retrospective effect law is not valid.

Rights of the accused during trial

There are numerous rights of defendant person in India approved once the trial is enduring in the court. The State has to ensure that due process of law is followed. The rights of the accused during the trial include the following:

- *Right to be examined by a medical practitioner:*
  - As requested by the arrested person so to do direct the examination of the body of such person by a registered physician if the magistrate considers that the appeal is made for the aim of deferring or for defeating the ends of justice. Section 54 (CrPC) elaborates the right as discussed.
- *Right to privacy and protection against unlawful searches:*
  - The privacy of the accused cannot be violated on a sheer assumption of a crime by the law officials. The property of an accused can be searched only with a search warrant by the officials.
- *Right to be present during trial:*
  - Section 273 of the Code makes it mandatory that the criminal lawyer or the accused must be present when each and every evidence and report are documented.
- *Right to get copies of documents:*
  - Copies of complete set of documents filed by the prosecutor pertinent to the case are shared with the accused.

- *Right to cross-examination:*
  - To establish the innocence of the accused, he or she has the right to be interrogated by the prosecuting attorney.
- *Right to appeal:*
  - Facilitates that a higher court can be appealed by the arrested citizen by filing a petition against his conviction.
- *Right to humane treatment in prison:*
  - The accused person when imprisoned should receive humane treatment by the prison authorities as a right and also should be assured all his human rights during the stay.
- *Right to be considered innocent till proven guilty:*
  - Until the guilt/crime is established by the court through evidences, the accused has the right to be considered innocent.

Post-trial rights of the accused person

The outcome of the trial determines if the accused person still has certain granted rights even after the trial is over. This concludes either he or she has been evidenced innocent by the court or has been held guilty and detained by law.

- **Rights of the accused, if declared innocent**

  When a person is declared innocent and not guilty by the court, the following rights are applicable:
  - Copy of the judgment is provided to the accused person.
  - The accused has the right to receive protection from police, if there are chances of threat to life after the trial.

Rights of the victim

'Victims' means persons who, individually or collectively, have suffered harm, including physical or mental injury, emotional suffering, economic loss or substantial impairment of their fundamental rights, through acts or omissions that are in violation of criminal laws operative within Member States, including those laws proscribing criminal abuse of power. This definition is endorsed by United Nations Human Rights.

The universal amendments grant the victims constitutional rights as follows:

Right to
- Fair treatment, with dignity and respect
- Notification of events/proceedings related to the trial
- Be present at the proceedings and trial
- Be granted restitution from an offender who is found guilty

Rights of the victims in India

The criminal justice system in India facilitates limited legal rights to be notified, present and heard to the victims. Court proceedings or the arrest or release of the defendant, are not to be notified to the victims. Victims do not have the right to be present for the trial or other proceedings, neither have they the rights to give a statement to the court at sentencing or at other hearings. Furthermore, victim assistance programmes are effectively nonexistent. The core rights of crime victims are presented in Fig. 4.2.

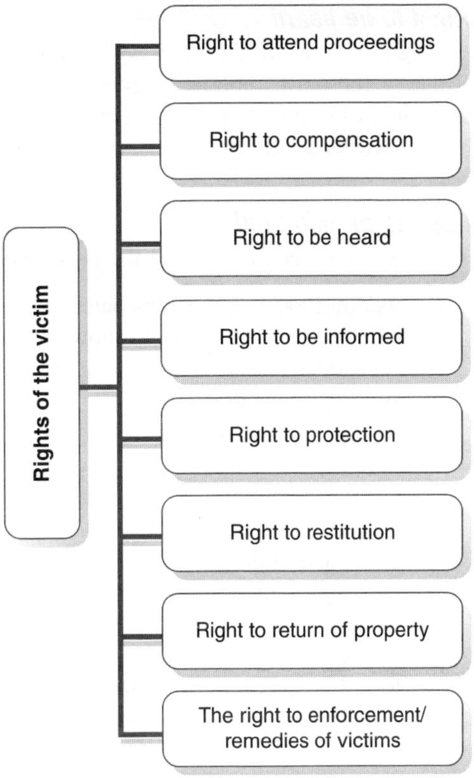

Fig. 4.2

Rights of the victim.

Right to attend proceedings

Criminal justice proceedings are allowed to be witnessed by crime victims and their families as a legal right. This right is important to victims, as it facilitates in observing the progression of the proceedings, to see the criminal justice process at work. The family and the victim can be part by listening to counsel's arguments, judge's viewpoint, witnesses and the defendant.

Attending trial, sentences and offender's bail hearing are the only rights given under this section to the victim; hence, the victim is not allowed to witness other proceedings. If the victim is a witness to the criminal case in such condition, he or she lacks the right to be present in such trials; this helps in averting the victim to be prejudiced after hearing the testimony of other case witnesses.

Furthermore, the victim of any crime is facilitated with the presence of an advocate or any member of the family during the proceedings of the case to support.

Right to compensation

The victim has the right to get reimbursement for the expenditures incurred pertinent to the crime, which is compensated through programmes under Government of India. This compensation amount is released from the state programme, i.e. same state of occurrence of the crime. The victim is compensated even if no individual is condemned for the crime or under arrest. Eligibility criteria for compensation are listed below.

COMPENSATION ELIGIBILITY

Victim who had reported the occurrence of the crime
Victim who liaised with the case trial
Person directly victimized of a vicious crime
Family of the demised victim
Victim of cases involving huge monetary cases
Medical/counselling/lawyer expenses of the victim
Paid back to people who help in settling the expenses of medical treatment/funeral of the victim
Victim/family should apply for compensation within stipulated time frame
Person is also compensated when there is loss in salary

Right to be heard

The right to be heard during grave criminal justice proceedings that impacts the welfare of the victim is one of the most important rights for crime victims. This helps them to participate actively in the procedure of criminal justice. The judiciary system acknowledges the statements/evidences submitted by the victims during the trial hearings.

Right to be informed

The victim and the family have the right to be updated about the following:

- Happenings/events/schedules/outcomes related to the case in which the victim is involved by the criminal justice system. The following events should always be informed:
    - Arrest/detention/custody of the accused
    - Hearing of the defendant
    - Release on bail and connected proceedings
    - Pretrial release and connected proceedings
    - Charge dismissal
    - Negotiated petitions and entry of petition bargain
    - Dates and timings of trials
    - Hearings related to sentencing
    - Concluding verdict/sentence or disposition
    - Probation or parole conditions
    - Relief proceedings of posttrials
    - Procedure for appeal and related proceedings
    - Parole release and related proceedings
    - Pardon/commutation of sentence and related proceedings
    - Cancellation, postponement and rescheduled dates are also updated to the victim
    - Final release from imprisonment, even if from a mental institution
    - Escape and ensuing rearrest of offender
- Legal rights of the victim are always notified:
    - Rights related to
        - attending a proceeding and/or submit a victim impact statement
        - taking legal action against the offender for incurred financial damages in the civil justice system
        - legal protection of the victim and family against the offender

Right to protection

It is the right of the victim of the crime to get protection amidst the legal criminal procedure. Explicit protective measures provided to the victims are as follows:

- Protection by police, while travelling to the court and back
- Facility of separate and protected waiting areas during the court hearings which are away and separate from other waiting areas
- Observe protection programmes
- At the time of relocation of residence
- Refusal of bail or bail release with explicit conditions

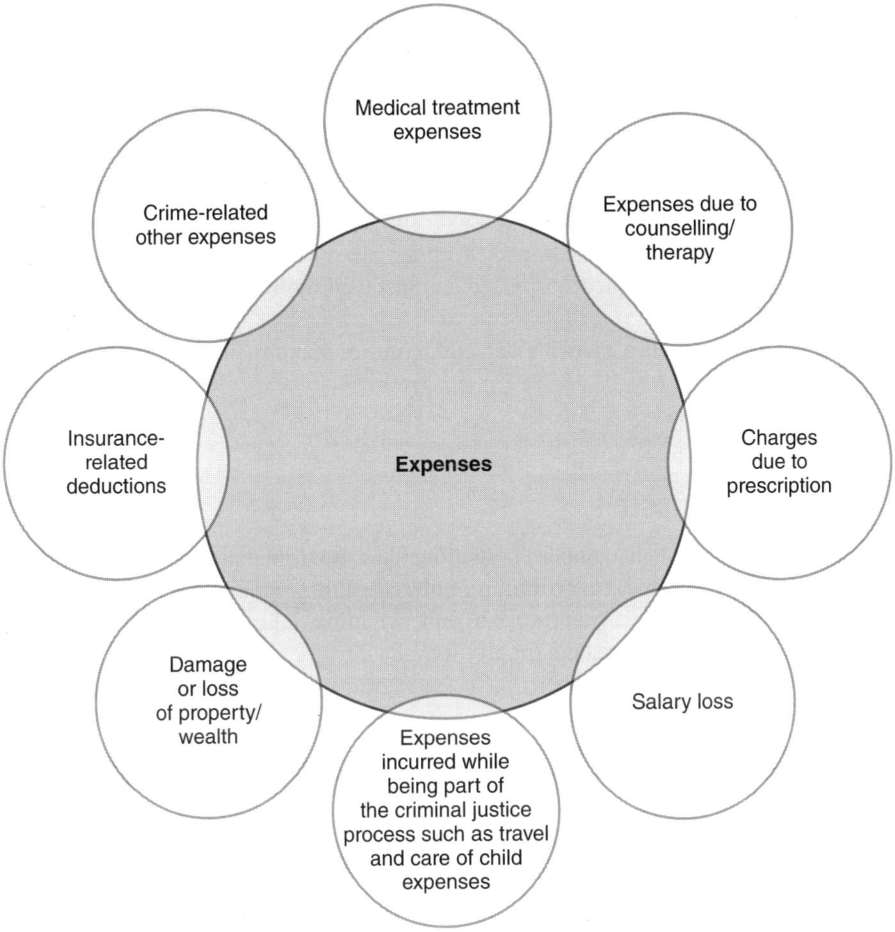

Fig. 4.3

Expenses compensated under right to restitution.

Right to restitution

Restoration of the damage/destruction done by the defendant, mostly in the form of compensation for damages is known 'restitution'. Details of losses that are out-of-pocket expenses which can be reimbursed pertinent to the crime are illustrated in Fig. 4.3.

Right to return of property

Robbery of property or when it is seized on lieu as proof/evidence for the case are the instances when a victim suffers a loss of property. The victim has the right to get back the property.

Right to a speedy trial

The victim of the crime is granted the right, wherein a speedy/promptness in the proceedings of the trial is done by avoiding arbitrary delays. Even though this right is granted, but it has limitations, as the numerous cases need time to be judged. In such cases, the victim has right to compensation/ restitution.

Right to enforcement/remedies of victims

Legal rights are granted to the victims by law, it is essential to confirm that those rights are enforced. There are few more other grants being given such as:

- Victim to pursue a writ of mandamus
- A court order engaged to an agency to obey with the law
- Complaints of the victim accepted, inspected and resolved by formation of a selected unit for this purpose
- An ombudsman or state victim advocate or a committee or board to provide remedy when the rights are violated

Human Rights Commission

Human rights have been established under international law as a foundation for public health, facilitating a basis for human rights awareness through public health practice over the last seven decades. Human rights provide a worldwide framework to enhance impartiality in public health, expanding the autonomies and powers needed to realize dignity for all.

Human Rights

Human rights are the basic rights of an individual, which are innate, integral and essential in one's nature irrespective of age, origin, geographic location, language, religious belief and cultural background (Table 4.3). These rights are societal norms and moral principles to maintain basic human behaviour and are often safeguarded by law. Human rights are universal and uniform and valid at all times for each individual. Human beings eventually lose their individuality and identity in the absence of the human rights. These rights are not applicable only in exceptional circumstances. These characteristic facets are endorsed by the United Nations.

Universal protection of the human rights as legal documents were undertaken by The Universal Declaration of Human Rights (UDHR), adopted by the United Nations General Assembly in 1948. This is the basis of all international human rights law and consists of 30 articles describing the principles, foundation of existing and upcoming human rights conventions, agreements and other legal entities.

Annually, 10 December is celebrated as Human Rights Day across the globe to commemorate the acceptance of UDHR by the UN General Assembly. The theme for year 2020 was 'Recover Better - Stand Up for Human Rights', which highlighted the COVID-19 pandemic and emphasized on the necessity to shape back or improve by confirming that human rights are pivotal to recovery efforts. Generating equivalent opportunities for all is the only way to achieve mutual global goals. The day marks the occasion to confirm the status of human rights in rebuilding the desired world, requirement for universal harmony as well as interrelation and collective human race. The theme helped to reinforce by engaging the common people/citizens, associates and the organization of UN to strengthen transformative acts that can help in improving and nurturing more resilient and unbiased societies.

Table 4.3 Human rights

Right to freedom from discrimination	*Right to life, freedom and personal security*	*Right to equality*	*Right to education*	*Freedom of opinion and information*
Right to marriage and family	*Freedom of belief and religion*	*Right to rest and leisure*	*Right to adequate living standard*	*Right to free ovement in and out of the country*
Right to equality before law	*Right to be considered innocent until proven guilty*	*Right to recognition as a person before the law*	*Right to appeal against legal decisions*	*Right to fair public hearing*
Freedom from torture and degrading Treatment	*Right to remedy by competent tribunal*	*Freedom from arbitrary arrest and exile*	*Right to participate in government and in free elections*	*Right to a nationality and the freedom to change it*
Right to participate in the cultural life of the community	*Right to gather for community activities*	*Right of peaceful assembly and association*	*Right to live in an orderly society*	*Right to desirable work and to join trade unions*
Freedom from state or personal interference in the above rights	*Freedom from slavery*	*Right to social security*	*Right to own property*	*Freedom from interference with privacy, family, home and correspondence*

Definitions

'Human rights are inherent to all human beings, regardless of race, sex, nationality, ethnicity, language, religion, or any other status'.

–United Nations Body

'Rights relating to life, liberty, equality and dignity of the individual guaranteed by the Constitution or embodied in the International Covenants and enforceable by courts in India'.

– Protection of Human Rights Act, India, Section 2(1)(d)

Salient features of human rights (Fig. 4.4)

1. Principle of Universality of human rights is the keystone pertinent to international human rights law. It implies each individual is equally eligible to the human rights. UDHR highlighted this principle as most important. It is mentioned frequently and constantly in various international human rights forums, conventions and resolutions.
2. Principle of Inalienability describes that the rights are applicable at all times and are withdrawn in exceptional circumstances and only after following a protocol/law. Examples:
   a. In case an individual is condemned by the court of law, then the right to liberty may be constrained.
   b. During COVID-19 pandemic, the human rights of the elderly living in old-age homes were jeopardized (Anand et al., 2021).
3. Principle of Indivisibility and Interdependency: This principle describes that the sets/clusters of rights can be enjoyed together.

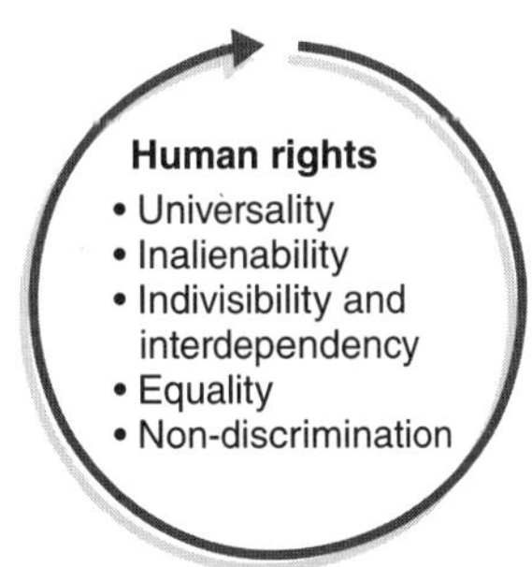
Human rights
• Universality
• Inalienability
• Indivisibility and interdependency
• Equality
• Non-discrimination

Fig. 4.4

Salient features of human rights.

In other words, it implies that violation of one set of rights may adversely/undesirably impact others.

4. Principle of Equality: This describes that each individual is born free by birth and is equivalent to other individuals in terms of dignity and rights. This is detailed by UDHR in Article 1.
5. Principle of Nondiscrimination, elaborated in Article 2 of UDHR, details about freedom from any kind of discrimination among the citizens and this further conforms and strengthens the principle of equality.

Similarities between human rights and fundamental rights

Human rights and fundamental rights are diverse in opinion of law, although there are few alike façades. The following are the similarities:

- The basic goal of both rights is to ensure individuals and the enforcement of agreeable and unbiased social law/order.
- Equipping citizens with ways of living and facilitating them to understand their maximum potential.
- Law and regulatory bodies help to support and sustain both the rights.
- Citizens are privileged with both the rights as the pivot of their lives.

Divergences between human rights and fundamental rights

There are few basic differences between both the rights despite the fact that they overlay each other very proximally (Table 4.4).

Human rights bodies

There are regulatory bodies at various levels that are responsible for promotion and protection of the human rights of citizens across the globe. The UN bodies are functional at the international level, whereas at country level there is National Human Rights Commission (NHRC) and further to this, each state of India has its State Human Rights Commission (SHRC) (Fig. 4.5).

Table 4.4 Differences between human rights and fundamental rights

Human rights	Fundamental rights
All human beings are eligible to experience these basic rights irrespective of the geographic location.	The citizens of a particular nation only can enjoy these basic rights and as put down by the constitution of that particular nation.
International Bill of Human Rights has the authority to outline these rights.	Constitution of the nation has the authority to outline these rights; hence, they differ nation to nation.
Universal rights are enjoyed equally across the globe.	Constitutional rights are unique to a specific country.
Regulatory bodies like United Nations and Human Rights Commission have the authority to frame and protect them.	Court of law is authorized to enforce them; hence, the citizen can approach the court of law in case of a breach in the rights and they are justifiable.

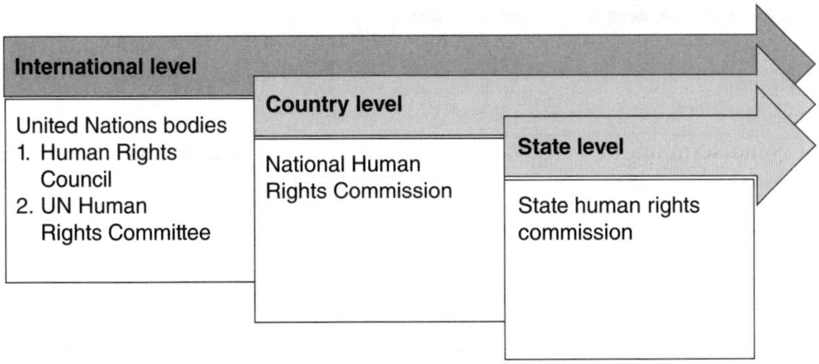

Fig. 4.5

Multilevelled human rights bodies.

United Nations Human Rights Council

The Human Rights Council is an intergovernmental body within the UN system accountable for the advancement and safety of all human rights worldwide. All thematic human rights issues and situations that require its attention throughout the year are addressed by the council.

The Council session is held annually at the UN Office at Geneva. Between mid-September to early October 2021, Human Rights Council conducted its 48th regular session, whereas its 31st special session was conducted in August 2021 addressing on the grave human rights concerns and situation in Afghanistan.

The Council comprises 47 Member States, which are elected by the majority of members of the General Assembly of the UN. India is member of the council. Equitable geographical distribution is the criteria for membership of the Council; the seats are distributed as follows:

1. African States: 13 seats
2. Asia-Pacific States: 13 seats
3. Latin American and Caribbean States: 8 seats
4. Western European and other States: 7 seats
5. Eastern European States: 6 seats

United Nations Human Rights Committee

The UN Human Rights Committee is a UN expert body composed of 18 experts founded by a human rights treaty known as the International Covenant on Civil and Political Rights (ICCPR). The committee meets annually, and discusses matters related to the aspects in the treaty.

The UN Human Rights Committee should not be confused with the more high-profile UN Human Rights Council, or its antecedent, the UN Commission on Human Rights. The Human Rights Council (since June 2006) and the Commission on Human Rights (before that date) are UN political bodies, composed of states, established by a UN General Assembly resolution and the UN Charter, and discussing the entire range of human rights concerns; the Human Rights Committee is a UN expert body, composed of persons, established by the ICCPR, and discussing matters pertaining only to that treaty.

Fundamental rights and freedom are protected by formation of the UN Commission on Human Rights in 1946.

Goals of the UN Human Rights Committee (Fig. 4.6)

Goals

- Governs the conduct of the citizens across the globe by establishing standards.
- Discourses the concerns pertinent to human rights.
- Protection of the fundamental rights of the special category of people:
  o The women, children, migrant workers, minorities and displaced persons.
- Scrutinize, monitor and publicly report
  - Either on human rights situations in specific countries or territories.
  - Or violation of human rights.
- Providing advisory services and technical cooperation related to human rights.

Fig. 4.6

Goals of the UN Human Rights Committee.

The National Human Rights Commission of India

NHRC is a self-governing, statutory public body constituted with the objective of protection and promotion of human rights of the Indian citizens at the national level. The headquarters of the Commission is located at New Delhi. NHRC looks over the rights that are related to life, dignity, liberty and equality of the individual that is defined in Section 2(1) of the Protection of Human Rights Act (PHRA). They are guaranteed by the Constitution of India, embodied in the international covenants and are enforceable by the courts of India as well.

Milestones towards formation of NHRC (Fig. 4.7)

The first milestone was achieved with the declaration of universal protection for human rights when UDHR was adopted by the UN General Assembly in Paris on 10 December 1948 (Table 4.5). Subsequently, the need was identified to strengthen the institutions of human rights at the national level, which led to the framing of an elaborate set of principles known as Paris Principles in 1991. Formation and functionality of numerous institutions were guided by the Paris Principles. Later in 1993, PHRA was passed to enhance the liability and strengths of the human rights in India. NHRC was founded in agreement with the Paris Principles, which were accepted for the promotion and protection of Human Rights and were sanctioned by the UN at its General Assembly of 1993.

Vision and mission

NHRC, India, has been constituted by an act of Parliament under PHRA 1993, with the vision of protection and advancement of human rights of Indian citizens. Section 12 of PHRA elaborates all the functions of the Commission. Its foremost and pivotal responsibility is to investigate or conduct enquiry pertinent to the human right violation grievances. Secondly, the commission proactively participates in creating human rights awareness amid the Indian citizens.

Mission of the Commission is to promote and protect human rights of each citizen of India and enhance the reach of Commission to the grassroots level, especially the weaker, neglected and disregarded societal strata.

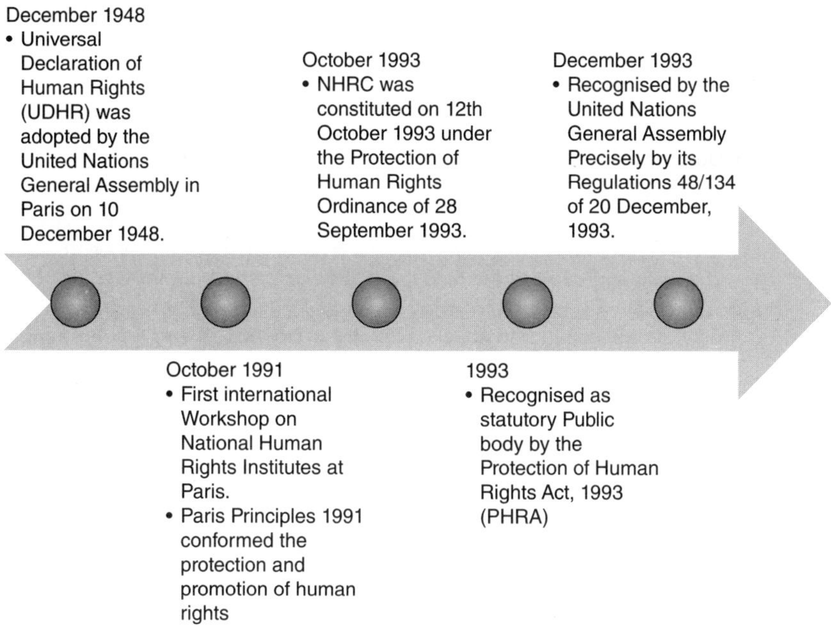

Fig. 4.7

NHRC development milestones.

Table 4.5 Universal Declaration of Human Rights

Article	Description
Article I	All human beings are born free and equal in dignity and rights. They are endowed with reason and conscience and should act towards one another in a spirit of brotherhood.
Article 2	Everyone is entitled to all the rights and freedoms set forth in this Declaration, without distinction of any kind, such as race, colour, sex, language, religion, political or other opinion, national or social origin, property, birth or other status. Furthermore, no distinction shall be made on the basis of the political, jurisdictional or international status of the country or territory to which a person belongs, whether it be independent, trust, non–self-governing or under any other limitation of sovereignty.
Article 3	Everyone has the right to life, liberty and security of person.
Article 4	No one shall be held in slavery or servitude; slavery and the slave trade shall be prohibited in all their forms.
Article 5	No one shall be subjected to torture or to cruel, inhuman or degrading treatment or punishment.
Article 6	Everyone has the right to recognition everywhere as a person before the law.
Article 7	All are equal before the law and are entitled without any discrimination to equal protection of the law. All are entitled to equal protection against any discrimination in violation of this Declaration and against any incitement to such discrimination.
Article 8	Everyone has the right to an effective remedy by the competent national tribunals for acts violating the fundamental rights granted him by the constitution or by law.
Article 9	No one shall be subjected to arbitrary arrest, detention or exile.
Article 10	Everyone is entitled in full equality to a fair and public hearing by an independent and impartial tribunal, in the determination of his rights and obligations and of any criminal charge against him or her.

Continued

Table 4.5 Universal Declaration of Human Rights—cont'd

Article	Description
Article 11	**1.** Everyone charged with a penal offence has the right to be presumed innocent until proved guilty according to law in a public trial at which he has had all the guarantees necessary for his or her defence. **2.** No one shall be held guilty of any penal offence on account of any act or omission which did not constitute a penal offence, under national or international law, at the time when it was committed. Nor shall a heavier penalty be imposed than the one that was applicable at the time the penal offence was committed.
Article 12	No one shall be subjected to arbitrary interference with his or her privacy, family, home or correspondence, nor to attacks upon his or her honour and reputation. Everyone has the right to the protection of the law against such interference or attacks.
Article 13	**1.** Everyone has the right to freedom of movement and residence within the borders of each State. **2.** Everyone has the right to leave any country, including his or her own, and to return to his or her country.
Article 14	**1.** Everyone has the right to seek and to enjoy in other countries asylum from persecution. **2.** This right may not be invoked in the case of prosecutions genuinely arising from nonpolitical crimes or from acts contrary to the purposes and principles of the United Nations.
Article 15	**1.** Everyone has the right to a nationality. **2.** No one shall be arbitrarily deprived of his nationality nor denied the right to change his or her nationality.
Article 16	**1.** Men and women of full age, without any limitation due to race, nationality or religion, have the right to marry and to found a family. They are entitled to equal rights as to marriage, during marriage and at its dissolution. **2.** Marriage shall be entered into only with the free and full consent of the intending spouses. **3.** The family is the natural and fundamental group unit of society and is entitled to protection by society and the State.
Article 17	**1.** Everyone has the right to own property alone as well as in association with others. **2.** No one shall be arbitrarily deprived of his or her property.
Article 18	Everyone has the right to freedom of thought, conscience and religion; this right includes freedom to change his religion or belief, and freedom, either alone or in community with others and in public or private, to manifest his religion or belief in teaching, practice, worship and observance.
Article 19	Everyone has the right to freedom of opinion and expression; this right includes freedom to hold opinions without interference and to seek, receive and impart information and ideas through any media and regardless of frontiers.
Article 20	**1.** Everyone has the right to freedom of peaceful assembly and association. **2.** No one may be compelled to belong to an association.
Article 21	**1.** Everyone has the right to take part in the government of his or her country, directly or through freely chosen representatives. **2.** Everyone has the right to equal access to public service in his country. **3.** The will of the people shall be the basis of the authority of government; this will shall be expressed in periodic and genuine elections which shall be held by universal and equal suffrage and shall be held by secret vote or by equivalent free voting procedures.

Table 4.5 Universal Declaration of Human Rights—cont'd

Article	Description
Article 22	Everyone, as a member of society, has the right to social security and is entitled to realization, through national effort and international cooperation and in accordance with the organization and resources of each State, of the economic, social and cultural rights indispensable for his or her dignity and the free development of his or her personality.
Article 23	**1.** Everyone has the right to work, to free choice of employment, to just and favourable conditions of work and to protection against unemployment. **2.** Everyone, without any discrimination, has the right to equal pay for equal work. **3.** Everyone who works has the right to just and favourable remuneration ensuring for himself or herself and his or her family an existence worthy of human dignity, and supplemented, if necessary, by other means of social protection. **4.** Everyone has the right to form and to join trade unions for the protection of his or her interests.
Article 24	Everyone has the right to rest and leisure, including reasonable limitation of working hours and periodic holidays with pay.
Article 25	**1.** Everyone has the right to a standard of living adequate for the health and well-being of himself or herself and of his or her family, including food, clothing, housing and medical care and necessary social services, and the right to security in the event of unemployment, sickness, disability, widowhood, old age or other lack of livelihood in circumstances beyond his or her control. **2.** Motherhood and childhood are entitled to special care and assistance. All children, whether born in or out of wedlock, shall enjoy the same social protection.
Article 26	**1.** Everyone has the right to education. Education shall be free, at least in the elementary and fundamental stages. Elementary education shall be compulsory. Technical and professional education shall be made generally available and higher education shall be equally accessible to all on the basis of merit. **2.** Education shall be directed to the full development of the human personality and to the strengthening of respect for human rights and fundamental freedoms. It shall promote understanding, tolerance and friendship among all nations, racial or religious groups, and shall further the activities of the United Nations for the maintenance of peace. **3.** Parents have a prior right to choose the kind of education that shall be given to their children.
Article 27	**1.** Everyone has the right to participate freely in the cultural life of the community, to enjoy the arts and to share in scientific advancement and its benefits. **2.** Everyone has the right to the protection of the moral and material interests resulting from any scientific, literary or artistic production of which he or she is the author.
Article 28	Everyone is entitled to a social and international order in which the rights and freedoms set forth in this Declaration can be fully realized.
Article 29	**1.** Everyone has duties to the community in which alone the free and full development of his or her personality is possible. **2.** In the exercise of his or her rights and freedoms, everyone shall be subject only to such limitations as are determined by law solely for the purpose of securing due recognition and respect for the rights and freedoms of others and of meeting the just requirements of morality, public order and the general welfare in a democratic society. **3.** These rights and freedoms may in no case be exercised contrary to the purposes and principles of the United Nations.
Article 30	Nothing in this Declaration may be interpreted as implying for any State, group or person any right to engage in any activity or to perform any act aimed at the destruction of any of the rights and freedoms set forth herein.

[Source: https://www.un.org/en/about-us/universal-declaration-of-human-rights]

NHRC, India, performs a dynamic responsibility in collaboration with other National Human Rights Institutes (NHRIs) across the globe with the perspective to augment cognizance related to human rights. It has also presented delegations to UN bodies and other NHRCs.

A former Chief Justice of India or a judge of the Supreme Court officiates as the Chairperson of the Commission; hence, NHRC is recognized as an exclusive institution with regard to employing robust monitoring and protection of human rights among all the NHRIs across the globe. Justice Shri Arun Kumar Mishra is the present chairperson of NHRC since 2 June 2021.

Evidences endorse that Indian Constitution establishes stronger examples in terms of safeguarding the rights of Indian citizens. Following are the reasons (Star and Bharadwaj, 2021).

- Vision and mission of Indian constitutional framework are unique and different from other countries.
- The Constitution of India can be revised/amended with ease and thus it can keep pace with dynamics of the norms of society.
- Our judiciary system adopts differing and innovative approaches to interpret the constitutional rights of citizens, which widens the scope of Constitution in terms of citizen's rights.

Attributes of Human Rights Commission

- Promotion and protection of human rights remain as a priority and an obligation.
- Comprises numerous decision-makers, who are working on either full-time or part-time basis.
- The core function of the commission is to perform investigations.
- The authority is vested on the commission to provide recommendations subsequent to the performance of investigation.

Functions of National Human Rights Commission

NHRC executes the functions as enforced by the PHRA (Fig. 4.8).

Functions of NHRC

- **Enquiring** proactively and on priority:
  - 1. Violations of human rights by government of India.
  - 2. Overlooking of such violation by a civil servant/official.
- **Protecting** the human rights of citizens.
- **Endorsing** remedial measures for effective implementation of human rights.
- **Appraising** various factors, (inclusive of acts of terrorism) that hinder the enjoyment of human rights and recommend appropriate remedial measures.
- **Studying** treaties and other international pacts pertinent to human rights and making suggestions for their efficacious execution.
- **Undertaking** or sponsoring research projects pertinent to human rights.
- **Visiting** to the jails and studying the condition of the inmates.
- **Engaging** in education related to human rights across all societal strata.
- **Helping** to spread awareness related to safety of rights through publications, and various media.
- **Encouraging** the voluntary work and related to human rights undertaken by various organisations and NGOs.
- **Reinforcing** the need for human rights protection.
- **Demanding** any document or record from any court or office related to the human rights.

Fig. 4.8

Functions of National Human Rights Commission.

Roles of National Human Rights Commission (Fig. 4.9)

Protection related role

- Looking for redressal
- Seeking remedies through courts, tribunals.
- Investigating individual complaints.
- Addressing public enquiry
- Safe guarding the human right protectors
- Reviewing the conditions in custody amenities.

Education related role

- Promoting public awareness through campaigns
- Training commoners as well as and NGOs, police, prisons officials, armed force, journalists and judiciary.
- Engaging in publications of projects.
- Encouraging initiatives undertaken by common public.
- Conducting seminars and workshops.
- Conducting media events, press release/conferences for propagation of awareness.

Research related role

- It conducts, facilitates research projects pertinent to human rights.
- Universities, technical institutions and non-governmental organizations are associated for human rights related research activities.
- Encourages youngsters to take part in its research work.
- Research activities are oriented towards developing data base, systems across India with the perspective to safe guard the human rights and fight against abuse of rights.
- Sponsors human rights related research work on fulfilment of the guidelines laid down by NHRC.

Fig. 4.9

Roles of National Human Rights Commission.

Members of National Human Rights Commission

Indian President along with the approval of a special committee can appoint the NHRC Chairperson and members of the Commission. The Committee comprises the members as shown in Fig. 4.10.

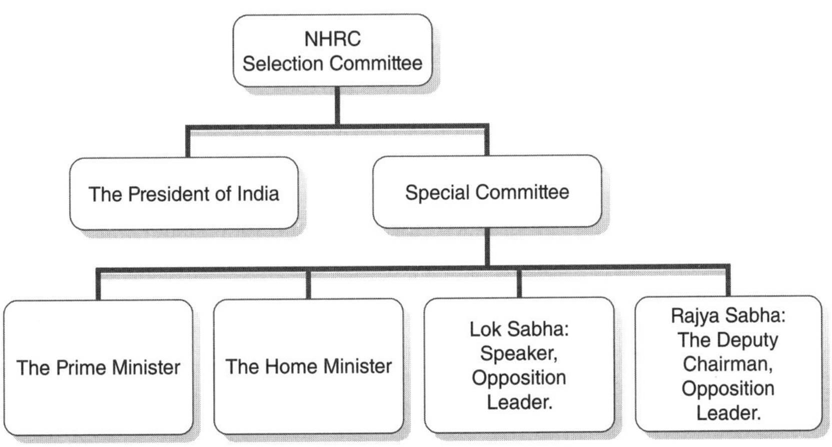

Fig. 4.10

NHRC selection committee.

Commission comprises the following nine members:

1. **Chairperson (1)**: A former Chief Justice of India or a Judge of the Supreme Court. Currently Justice Shri Arun Kumar Mishra is the officiating Chairperson.
2. **Member (1)**: Former or present Judge of the Supreme Court of India or Chief Justice of a High Court. Chief Justice of the Supreme Court has only the authority to suggest the appointment of these two members.
3. **Remaining three members:**
   a. Appointed members should be experienced and cognizant about issues related to human rights.
   b. At least one of them should be a female member.
4. **Ex-officio/deemed members (4):** Chairperson of following Commissions:
   a. National Commission for Minorities
   b. National Commission for Scheduled Castes
   c. National Commission for Scheduled Tribes
   d. National Commission for Women

Activities performed by National Human Rights Commission

1. Strategic planning
   a. Complaints and redressal mechanism
   b. Awareness raising, human rights education, training and research.
   c. Cooperation with all SHRCs and other national commissions
   d. Cooperation with civil society, NGOs and Human Rights Defenders
   e. Recognizing and protecting human rights defenders (Bennett, 2015)
   f. Monitoring and progress
   g. Engagement in international and regional bodies and mechanisms
2. Preparation and execution of annual action plan aligned with NHRC Strategic Plan 2018–2021 and the Sustainable Development Goals
3. Preparation of an annual budget
4. Conducting conferences, events on and meetings on regular basis

Challenges of National Human Rights Commission

- Subsequent recommendations of NHRC are not mandatory.
- NHRC jurisdiction does not include violation of the rights by private parties.
- NHRC does not have the authority to punish the systems that do not comply with its suggested instructions.
- Judicial perspective is added and highlighted in Commission functionality, as three of the NHRC members are judges.
- Cases related to army personnel are not judged by the Commission.
- NHRC faces challenges like overburden of cases, scarce resources, administrative delays, etc.
- Following cases are not included under NHRC jurisdiction:
  - Pending cases of more than 365 days
  - Unidentified, pseudonymous or vague cases
  - Cases which are trivial in nature
  - Service matters related cases

State Human Rights Commission

PHRA sanctioned the State Governments to create SHRC. This state commission has the authority to implement the powers deliberated upon, and to execute the functions assigned to it. Currently in India, there are 26 states with their own functional State Commissions, except the states of Arunachal Pradesh, Nagaland and Mizoram. West Bengal Human Rights Commission was the first to be constituted in 1994 at Kolkata whereas the latest one was constituted in 2019 as the Telangana SHRC. Discussed below is an example of SHRC functional in the state of Maharashtra:

- It was established in 2000 and subsequently was operational from next year March.
- It is located at Mumbai.
- A retired Chief Justice of the High Court officiates as the Chairperson.
- The number of members is two after an amendment in 2006.

Functions of State Human Rights Commission

- To investigate human rights violation/abuse or neglect in the stoppage of such violation by an administrator.
- To monitor state jails and detention places of convicts so as to study the staying condition and suggest improvements.
- To assess various aspects like terrorist activity within the state that hinder availing human rights and recommend appropriate remedial measures.
- To analyse the constitutional and other legal safeguards for the protection of human rights and discuss measures for their effective execution
- To conduct and sponsor research activities within the state, pertinent to human rights.
- To promote awareness about human rights amongst the commoners in the respective state and also to let people know about the safety measures existing for the protection of human rights.

Conclusion

Nursing professionals play varied proficient roles, one such role being the advocate for the patient. This chapter has brought in all the information pertinent to Indian Constitution, Fundamental Rights and exclusively the rights of an accused and the rights of the victim. Cognizance about these topics as a part of Forensic Nursing curriculum will enable the professionals to help the patient in a comprehensive manner, facilitating them to be aware of their basic rights when they are violated.

Multiple choice questions

1. **Who is considered as the father of Indian Constitution?**
   a. Dr B R Ambedkar
   b. Dr Rajendra Prasad
   c. Sardar Patel
   d. Maulana Azad

2. According to Indian Constitution there are _____ fundamental rights.
- a. 3
- b. 6
- c. 9
- d. 12

3. Restoration of the damage/destruction done by the defendant, mostly in the form of compensation for damages is called
- a. right to restitution
- b. right to protection
- c. right to be heard
- d. right to be informed

4. Which of the following is a fundamental right?
- a. Right to equality
- b. Right to freedom
- c. Right against exploitation
- d. All of the above

5. The Constitution of India came into force in
- a. 1950
- b. 1947
- c. 1948
- d. 1949

Further reading

1. Bakshi PM, Kashyap SC. *The Constitution of India*. New Delhi: Universal Law Publishing; 1982.
2. Basu DD, Manohar VR, Banerjee BP, Khan SA. *Introduction to the Constitution of India*. New Delhi: Wadhwa; 2001.
3. Singh DK, Shukla VN. *The Constitution of India*. Lucknow: Eastern Book Company; 1975.
4. Sharma BK. *Introduction to the Constitution of India*. New Delhi: PHI Learning Pvt. Ltd.; 2021.
5. Merillat HC. *Land and the Constitution in India*. Bombay: NM Tripathi; 1970.
6. Dash SC. *The Constitution of India. A Comparative Study*. Allahabad: Chaitanya Publishing House; 1968.
7. Singh MP, Deva S. The constitution of India: symbol of unity in diversity. *Jahrbuch des Offentlichen Rechts der Gegenwart, Yearb Public Law (Germany)*. 2005;53:649-686.
8. Sripati V. Toward fifty years of constitutionalism and fundamental rights in India: looking back to see ahead (1950-2000). *Am Univ Int Law Rev*. 1998;14:413.
9. De Villiers B. Directive principles of state policy and fundamental rights: the Indian experience. *S Afr J Hum Rights*. 1992;8(1):29-49.
10. Ready SS. Fundamentalness of fundamental rights and directive principles in the Indian Constitution. *J Indian Law Inst*. 1980;22(3):399-407.
11. Jain T. *Influence of Universal Declaration on the Judicial Interpretation of Fundamental Rights and Directive Principles in the Constitution of India*. Available at: SSRN 1087594. 2004, December 1.
12. Subbarao GC. Fundamental rights in India versus power to amend the constitution. *Tex Int'l LF*. 1968;4:291.
13. RC. Constitutional Law—Right to Equality—Discrimination in Transfer of income-tax cases—S. 5 (7A) of Indian Income-tax Act, 1922 vis-a-vis Article 14 of the Constitution of India. *J Indian Law Inst*. 1959;1:300-307.
14. Kashyap SC. Constitution of India and International Law. In: Patel BN, ed. *India and International Law*; 2005 Jan 1 (pp. 9-32). Leiden/Boston: Brill Nijhoff.
15. Johari JC. *The Constitution of India a Politico-legal Study*. New Delhi: Sterling Publishers Pvt. Ltd; 2007.
16. Ghosh PK. *The Constitution of India—How it has been Framed.* Calcutta: World Press; 1966; 427.

17. Singh MP, Deva S. The constitution of India: symbol of unity in diversity. *Jahrbuch des Offentlichen Rechts der Gegenwart, Yearb Public Law (Germany)*. 2005;53:649-686.
18. Krishnakumar T. Law enforcement access to data in India: considering the past, present, and future of section 91 of the code of criminal procedure, 1973. *Indian J Law Tech*. 2019;15:67.
19. Moore, S.A., Faulkner, G., Rhodes, R.E. et al. Impact of the COVID-19 virus outbreak on movement and play behaviours of Canadian children and youth: a national survey. Int J Behav Nutr Phys Act 17, 85 (2020). https://doi.org/10.1186/s12966-020-00987-8
20. Human Rights Day. https://www.un.org/en/observances/human-rights-day
21. United Nations Human Rights council. https://www.ohchr.org/en/hrbodies/chr/pages/commissiononhumanrights.aspx
22. National Human Rights Commission India https://nhrc.nic.in/about-us/about-the-Organisation.
23. What are human rights? https://www.ohchr.org/en/issues/pages/whatarehumanrights.aspx.
24. Human Rights Body. https://www.ohchr.org/EN/HRBodies/Pages/HumanRightsBodies.aspx https://www.ohchr.org/EN/HRBodies/HRC/RegularSessions/Session48/Pages/48RegularSession.aspx https://www.ohchr.org/EN/HRBodies/HRC/SpecialSessions/Pages/SpecialSessions.aspx https://www.ohchr.org/EN/HRBodies/CHR/Pages/Background.aspx
25. National Human Rights Commission. About the Organisation. https://nhrc.nic.in/about-us/about-the-Organisation
26. Vision and Mission https://nhrc.nic.in/about-us/vision-and-mission
27. Research guidelines. https://nhrc.nic.in/training-&-research/research-studies-&-projects/research-guidelinesss
28. Membership of the Human Rights Council. https://www.ohchr.org/EN/HRBodies/HRC/Pages/Membership.aspx
29. Composition of the Commission. https://nhrc.nic.in/about-us/composition-of-commission http://hrlibrary.umn.edu/edumat/hreduseries/hereandnow/Part-5/8_udhr-abbr.htm
30. Universal declaration of human rights. https://www.un.org/en/about-us/universal-declaration-of-human-rights.
31. State Human Rights Commission. https://web.archive.org/web/20151208063348/http://www.nhrc.nic.in/shrc.htm

Research references

1. Anand JC, Donnelly S, Milne A, Nelson-Becker H, Vingare EL, Deusdad B, et al. The covid-19 pandemic and care homes for older people in Europe - deaths, damage and violations of human rights. European Journal of Social Work [Internet]. 2021;0(0):1–12. Available from: https://doi.org/10.1080/13691457.2021.1954886
2. Star S, Bharadwaj A. Constitutional rights and guarantees: the contrasting approaches of Australia and India. International Journal of Human Rights. 2021;13642987.
3. Bennett K, Ingleton D, Nah AM, Savage J. Critical perspectives on the security and protection of human rights defenders. International Journal of Human Rights. 2015;19(7):883–95.

UNIT

INDIAN JUDICIAL SYSTEM AND LAWS RELATED TO NURSING PRACTICE

V

Vikas P. Meshram and Tanuj Kanchan

Learning objectives

On completion of this chapter, the readers will be able to:

1. Explain Indian judicial system and laws.
2. Discuss the importance of POCSO Act.
3. Explicate in depth the basic concepts pertinent to Human Rights.
4. Enlist the salient features of Human Rights.
5. Identify the similarities and difference between Human Rights and Fundamental Rights.
6. Enlist the Human Rights.
7. Describe the Human Rights Bodies at various levels.
8. Explain about vision and mission of Human Rights Commission.
9. Elucidate in detail about functions, roles and activities of Human Rights Commission.
10. Enumerate about the members forming the Commission.

Indian judicial system

The Constitution of India divides the Indian judiciary into superior judiciary (the Supreme Court and the high courts) and the subordinate judiciary (the lower courts under the control of the high courts). Each state has one high court, although some high courts have jurisdiction over multiple states and union territories. For example, the Guwahati High Court exercises jurisdiction over the states of Assam, Nagaland, Mizoram and Arunachal Pradesh, all of which are situated close to each other in the northeastern part of India. For administrative convenience, states are further subdivided into districts, each of which has its own district court.

Structure or hierarchy of Indian judicial system

The judiciary in India has a hierarchical structure with the Supreme Court at the top followed by high courts and below them the district courts. The lower courts function under the direct superintendence of the higher courts (Fig. 5.1).

Supreme Court: It is also known as the apex court. It is the highest judicial tribunal and the last appellate court in India. It is located in New Delhi. It is presided by the Chief Justice of India. Usually, Supreme Court hears appeals against high court orders. However, it also takes up writ petitions regarding matters concerning serious human rights violations, constitutional rights, etc. Any order passed by Supreme Court is binding for all the lower courts.

High courts: These are the highest courts in the states and union territories. A high court is presided by its Chief Justice. The President of India appoints judges of a high court in consultation with the Chief Justice of India, Chief Justice of the high court and the Governor of the state. High court can try any offence and pass any sentence authorized by law.

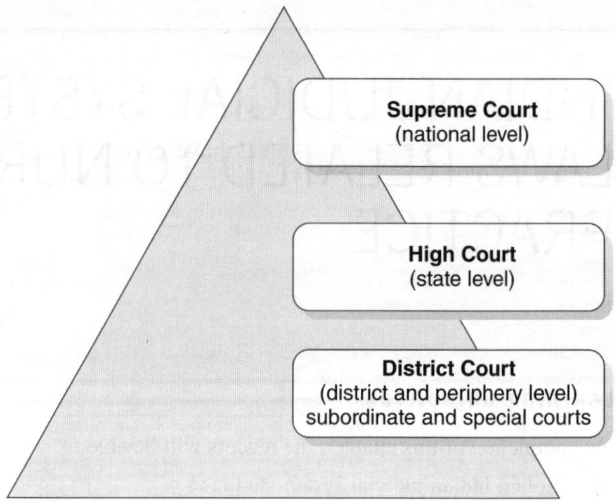

Fig. 5.1

Hierarchy of Indian judicial system.

District courts: These are established by the state governments of India for every district. It may cover one or more districts too, depending on the population and/or the number of cases. The district court is presided over by a District Judge appointed by the Governor of the state with the consultation of the high court. There can be Additional District Judges and Assistant District Judges depending on the workload. These courts can deal with serious offences, i.e. those carrying a punishment of imprisonment of more than 7 years, life imprisonment or death. It can pass any sentence authorized by law, but the death penalty must be confirmed by high court.

There are certain subordinate courts or specialized courts at the district level which consider both criminal cases and civil cases.

- **Magistrate courts:** Courts of the judicial magistrate are at lowest level of the Criminal Court structure in India. Magistrate is a lower post in the hierarchy than a judge. Magistrates are appointed by high court. In India, magistrates are of three types.
  - *Chief judicial magistrate* can award a sentence of imprisonment up to 7 years and an unlimited fine.
  - *First class judicial magistrate* can award a sentence of imprisonment up to 3 years and a fine of Rs 10000.
  - *Second class judicial magistrate* can award a sentence of imprisonment up to 1 year and a fine of Rs 5000.

  In metropolitan cities with more than 1 million, chief judicial magistrate and first class judicial magistrate are designated as *chief metropolitan magistrate* and *metropolitan magistrate*, respectively.
- **Juvenile court:** These are courts for the trial of children under the age of 18 years who are in conflict with the law or in need of care and protection. The purpose of a separate court is sociolegal rehabilitation and reformation, not punishment. This court is presided by first class woman magistrate.
- **Consumer court:** These are special types of courts that deal with consumer-related disputes regarding any goods or services. A consumer can claim compensation in these courts. According to the level of compensation, the claim can be made to the district forum (up to Rs 20 lakhs), state

forum (Rs 20 lakhs to 1 crore) and national forum (more than Rs 1 crore). Supreme Court is the last appellate court for appeal against the decision of the national forum. Medical services also come under the ambit of the Consumer Protection Act, except when all the hospital services are provided free of cost at all the times.

- **Family courts:** District courts have certain traditional courts which are formed under specific statues. For example, family courts deal with issues related to marriage, guardianship of minors, etc.
- **Specialized courts:** There are certain local bodies for the Indian judicial system at the periphery level such as *Lok Adalats* and *Gram Panchayats* to settle the local disputes. Additionally, there are quasijudicial to oversee the specific legal problems and to deal with specific statutes. For example, the Central Administrative Tribunal has been established to settle the disputes and complaints with respect to the recruitment and conditions of service of persons appointed to public services. The National Human Rights Commission (NHRC) of India is a statutory public body for the protection of human rights.

Functions of the Indian judicial system

1. **Protection of the fundamental rights of the citizen:** The judiciary system has the power to ensure justice when there is any violation of fundamental rights of any citizen.
2. **Protection of the Constitution of India:** The Supreme Court acts as the guardian of the Constitution of India. The conflicts of jurisdiction between the central government and the state governments or between the legislature and the executive are decided by the court.
3. **Administration of justice:** The chief function of the judiciary system is the proper enactment of the law to ensure justice.
4. **Supervisory functions:** The higher courts have the function of supervising the subordinate courts in India.
5. **Advisory functions:** The Supreme Court in India performs an advisory function during situations such as inappropriate indulgent in the constitution of India by central government and the state governments

Indian judiciary system – laws

India has a single integrated judicial system in which there are two branches for the legal system.

- **Criminal law:** It deals with the legal proceedings related to the crime committed by any citizen of India. The examples for the violation of the criminal laws are murder, robbery, etc.
- **Civil law:** It deals with the disputes related to the violation of the fundamental rights of a citizen. The examples for the violation of the civil laws are divorce, consumer problems, etc.

Major sources of law in India

The major domestic sources of law are as follows:

- **The Constitution of India:** The supreme source of law in India is the Constitution of India which contains 395 articles in 22 parts. This is a document that provides a framework for the fundamental political code, structure, procedures, powers and duties of government institutions and fundamental rights, directive principles and the duties of citizens. It was adopted by the Constituent Assembly of India on 26 November 1949 and became effective on 26 January 1950.

- **Statutes:** Statutes are the written laws enacted by the Parliament or the state legislatures. At the local level, these legislations are passed by local authorities such as government departments, municipal corporations, etc.
- **Customary law:** The customary laws are the information regarding the customs and traditional practices observed in a particular community or society. The local customs that are not against any statute or morality are considered while drafting certain laws (usually religious in nature).
- **Judicial decisions:** The judicial opinion is a form of legal opinion written by a judge or a judicial panel in the course of resolving a legal dispute. The judicial decisions of superior courts like the Supreme Court of India and high courts are another important legal source of laws.

Laws – civil and criminal case procedures

Indian judicial procedures are usually governed by the Indian Penal Code, Criminal Procedure Code and Indian Evidence Act.

Indian Penal Code

The Indian Penal Code (IPC) is the official criminal code of India. It is a comprehensive code consisting of 511 sections intended to cover all substantive aspects of criminal law. The list of IPCs related to the medical profession is listed below.

Sections related to consent

Section	Content
Section 87 of IPC	Act not intended and not known to be likely to cause death or grievous hurt, done by consent
Section 88 of IPC	Act not intended to cause death, done by consent in good faith for person's benefit
Section 89 of IPC	Act done in good faith for the benefit of a child or insane person, by or by consent of the guardian
Section 90 of IPC	Consent known to be given under fear or misconception
Section 92 of IPC	Act done in good faith for the benefit of a person without consent

Section related to medical negligence

Section	Content
Section 304 A of IPC	Causing death by rash or negligent act
Section 336 of IPC	Committing rash or negligent act endangering life or personal safety of others
Section 337 of IPC	Causing hurt by rash or negligent act endangering life or personal safety of others
Section 338 of IPC	Causing grievous hurt by rash or negligent act endangering life or personal safety of others

Section related to intimation to police and evidence preservation in medicolegal cases

Section	Content
Section 176 of IPC	Omission to give notice or information to public servant by person legally bound to give it
Section 177 of IPC	Furnishing false information
Section 201 of IPC	Causing disappearance of evidence of the offence or giving false information to screen offender
Section 202 of IPC	Intentional omission to give information about offence by person bound to inform

Sections related to medicolegal aspects of wound

Section	Content
Section 44 of IPC	Legal definition of injury
Section 299 of IPC	Culpable homicide
Section 300 of IPC	Murder
Section 302 of IPC	Punishment for murder
Section 304 of IPC	Punishment for culpable homicide not amounting to murder
Section 304 B of IPC	Dowry death
Section 306 of IPC	Abetment of suicide
Section 307 of IPC	Attempt to murder
Section 319 of IPC	Hurt
Section 320 of IPC	Grievous hurt
Section 323 and 325 of IPC	Punishment for voluntary causing hurt and grievous hurt
Section 324 and 326 of IPC	Punishment for voluntary causing hurt and grievous hurt by dangerous weapons or means
Section 326 A and 326 B of IPC	Voluntary causing grievous hurt by acid or other corrosive substance

Sections related to sexual offences

Section	Content
Section 166B of IPC	Punishment for failure to provide first aid or medical treatment free of cost and mandatory information to police (imprisonment for 1 year)
Section 228A of IPC	Punishment for revealing the identity of survivor of rape (imprisonment for 2 years)
Section 354 of IPC	Assault or criminal force to woman with intent to outrage her modesty (imprisonment for 2 years)
Section 354A of IPC	Sexual harassment (imprisonment for 1–3 years)
Section 354B of IPC	Assault or use of criminal force with intent to disrobe (imprisonment for 3–7 years)
Section 354C of IPC	Voyeurism (imprisonment for 1–3 years and 3–7 years for subsequent offence)
Section 354D of IPC	Stalking (imprisonment for 3–5 years)
Section 375 of IPC	Rape
Section 376 of IPC and 376A to 376E	Punishment of rape (minimum imprisonment for 7 years and death penalty can also be awarded in certain offences)
Section 377 of IPC	Unnatural sexual offences (imprisonment for 10 years)

Criminal Procedure Code

It is also referred to as the Code of Criminal Procedure (CrPC). It was enacted in 1973. It is the main legislation for the procedure of administration of criminal laws in India. It provides a framework related to the criminal investigation, evidence collection, arrest of the suspect/accused, court procedure and punishment, etc. It consists of a total of 565 sections. Some of the relevant Criminal Procedure Codes related to the medical profession are listed below.

Section	Content
Section 39 of CrPC	Public to give information of certain offences
Section 53 of CrPC	Examination of accused by medical practitioner at the request of the police officer
Section 164A of CrPC	Medical examination of the victim of rape
Section 174 of CrPC	Police inquest into cause of death
Section 176 of CrPC	Magistrate inquest into cause of death

Indian Evidence Act

Indian Evidence Act was enacted in 1872. It provides a set of rules regarding the admissibility of evidence in the Court of law. The Act consists of 3 parts and 11 chapters. It broadly deals with the relevancy of the facts, the definition of an expert witness, oral evidence, documentary evidence, examination of the witnesses, etc.

Prevention of Children from Sexual Offences Act 2012 (POCSO Act 2012)

POCSO Act came into existence on 19 June 2012 in India. The act is to protect the children from offences of sexual assault, sexual harassment, pornography and also have the provision of special courts for trial of such offences. It is a gender-neutral act and is applicable to individuals younger than 18 years. Prior to this Act, sexual offences against male children were mostly covered under the ambit of section 377 of IPC, which defines unnatural sexual offences.

As per POCSO Act 2012, the sexual offences are classified into the following sections:

I. **Penetrative sexual assault (Section 3)**

A man is said to commit penetrative sexual assault

1. If he inserts his penis to any extent in the mouth, vagina, urethra or anus of the child or makes the child do so with him or any other person; or
2. If he inserts any object or any other body part, not being penis in the vagina, urethra or anus of the child or make the child does so with him or any other person; or
3. If he manipulates any part of the body of the child to cause penetration into vagina, urethra, anus or of any part of the body of the child or make the child does so with him or any other person; or
4. If he applies a mouth to the penis, vagina, urethra or anus of the child or make the child does so with him or any other person.

Punishment for this offence is 7 years of imprisonment and can be extended to life imprisonment (Section 4).

II. Aggravated penetrative sexual assault (Section 5)

Aggravated penetrative sexual assault is considered a more grave offence. It covers:

1. Penetrative sexual assault by the person in the position of authority. These personnel can be police officers, members of armed forces, public servants, management or staff of jail, remand home, protection home, observation home or any other place of custody, management or staff of hospital or management or staff of any educational or religious institution.
2. Gang penetrative sexual assault involving two or more perpetrators.
3. Penetrative sexual assault causing grievous injury or bodily harm or injury to the sexual organs of the child.
4. Penetrative sexual assault using a deadly weapon, fire, heated substance or corrosive substance.
5. Penetrative sexual assault causing grievous hurt or injury to the sex organ of the child.
6. Penetrative sexual assault causing physical or mental incapacitation.
7. Penetrative sexual assault causing pregnancy.
8. Penetrative sexual assault causing HIV transmission or any other life-threatening infection or disease.
9. Penetrative sexual assault is committed taking advantage of a child's mental or physical disability.
10. Penetrative sexual assault is committed more than once or repeatedly.
11. Penetrative sexual assault with a child younger 12 years.
12. When the perpetrator is a relative of the child.
13. When perpetrator commits offence on a child knowing the child is pregnant.
14. When an attempt is also made to murder the child.
15. When an offence is committed by a previous convict of a similar offence.
16. When an offence is committed, and a child is made to strip and/or paraded naked in public.
17. When an offence is committed in the course of communal or sectarian violence.

Punishment for this offence is 10 years of imprisonment and can be extended to life imprisonment (Section 6).

Additional sections of IPC can also be imposed in certain scenarios like:

a) Gang rape on woman under 16 years of age is punishable with imprisonment for the remainder of a person's natural life (376DA of IPC)
b) Gang rape on woman under 12 years of age is punishable with imprisonment for the remainder of a person's natural life or with the death penalty (376DB of IPC)
c) In cases of a person committing rape on a woman under 12 years of age, there is a provision of rigorous imprisonment for 20 years which can be extended to imprisonment for the remainder of a person's natural life with a fine or with the death penalty (376AB of IPC).

III. Sexual assault (Section 7)

Whoever with sexual intent touches the vagina, penis, anus or breast of the child or makes the child touch the vagina, penis, anus or breast of such person or any other person, or does any other act with sexual intent which involves physical contact without penetration is said to commit sexual assault. Punishment for this offence is 3–5 years of imprisonment (Section 8).

IV. Aggravated sexual assault (Section 9)

Sexual assault is considered aggravated in similar scenarios as described under Section 5, except the nature of sexual act does not result in pregnancy. Punishment for this offence is 5–7 years of imprisonment (Section 10).

V. Sexual harassment (Section 11)

A person is said to commit sexual harassment upon a child when such person with sexual intent,

1. Utters any word or makes any sound, or makes any gesture or exhibits any object or part of the body with the intention that such word or sound shall be heard, or such gesture or object or part of the body shall be seen by the child; or
2. Makes a child exhibit his or her body or any part of his or her body so as it is seen by such person or any other person; or
3. Shows any object to a child in any form or media for pornographic purposes; or
4. Repeatedly or constantly follows or watches or contacts a child either directly or through electronic, digital or any other means; or
5. Threatens to use, in any form of media, a real or fabricated depiction through electronic, film or digital or any other mode, of any part of the body of the child or the involvement of the child in a sexual act; or
6. Entices a child for pornographic purposes or gives gratification therefore.

Punishment for this offence is 3 years of imprisonment (Section 12).

Medical examination of child

- Section 27 of the POCSO Act covers the procedure for medical examination of the child in such offences. The examination is to be done in accordance with 164A CrPC.
- This Act mandates the examination of a girl child by a female registered medical practitioner. Examination of the child has to be carried out in the presence of the parent, guardian or any other person in whom the child deposes his or her trust.
- In the absence of any such person, an examination shall be conducted in the presence of a woman nominated by the head of the medical institution.

It is mandatory for a medical practitioner or any other person having knowledge about the commission of the offence under this Act to inform to police. Failure to do so can attract the punishment of 6 months of imprisonment. This Act strictly prohibits revealing the identity of a child in any sort of medium. The trial under this Act is in camera in the presence of a parent or any other person in whom the child deposes trust or confidence.

This Act emphasizes on child-friendly mechanisms like provision of the special juvenile police unit, recording of evidence at the place of choice of the child, the police officer should not be in the uniform while recording the statement, a child shall not come in contact with the accused, a child shall not to be a detained in a police station in the night and speedy trial of offences through designated special courts.

Multiple choice questions

1. The judges of the high court are appointed by
   a. President of India
   b. Chief Justice of India
   c. Prime Minister of India
   d. Union Minister of Law and Justice

2. The retirement age of the judges of a Supreme Court is
   a. 60 Years
   b. 62 Years
   c. 65 Years
   d. 75 Years
3. The retirement age of the judges of a high court is
   a. 60 Years
   b. 62 Years
   c. 65 Years
   d. 75 Years
4. Total number of high courts in India as of 2022 is
   a. 18
   b. 20
   c. 21
   d. 25
5. The ultimate power of interpreting the Constitution of India lies with
   a. Supreme Court of India
   b. High courts of India
   c. Session courts of India
   d. District courts of India
6. Prevention of Children from Sexual Offences Act came into existence in
   a. 2010
   b. 2011
   c. 2012
   d. 2013

Further Reading

1. Jois R. *Legal and Constitutional History of India: Ancient, Judicial and Constitutional System*. New Delhi: Universal Law Publishing; 2004.
2. Kumar R. *Universal's Guide to the Constitution of India*. New Delhi: Universal Law Publishing; 2011.
3. Saha TK. *Textbook on Legal Methods, Legal Systems and Research*. New Delhi:Universal Law Publishing; 2010.
4. Kansas. *The Code of Civil Procedure*. New Delhi: Universal Law Publishing; 1950.
5. Choudhry S, Khosla M, Mehta PB, eds. *The Oxford Handbook of the Indian Constitution*. Oxford, UK: Oxford University Press; 2016.
6. Minattur J, ed. *The Indian Legal System*. Mumbai: NM Tripathi Pvt Ltd; 1978.
7. Baxi U. Who bothers about the Supreme Court? The problem of impact of judicial decisions. *J Indian Law Inst*. 1982;24(4):848-862.
8. Sinha M. Land, Law and Courts in India: tracing land rights debates through processes of judicial decision making. *Dev Change*. 2019;50(4):1063-1082.
9. Vishwakarma S. The scope of changes in the criminal law system in India: to eradicate the non-effective provision in statue. *LingCuRe*. 2021;5(S4):2457-2469.
10. Austin G. *The Indian Constitution: Cornerstone of a Nation*. New Delhi: Oxford University Press; 1999.
11. Stephen JF. *The Indian Evidence Act (I. of 1872): With an Introduction on the Principles of Judicial Evidence*. London: Macmillan and Company; 1872.
12. Pande DC. *A Textbook on the Criminal Procedure Code*. New Delhi: Indian Law Institute; 1973.
13. Gaur KD. *Textbook on the Indian Penal Code*. New Delhi: Universal Law Publishing; 2009.

14. Chaudhary BL, Kr R. Medical examination of child of sexual assault under the protection of children from sexual offences (POSCO), act 2012. *IP Int J Forensic Med Toxicol Sci*. 2021;2(3):50-53.
15. Kshirsagar J. POCSO-an effective act of the era. *Supremo Amicus*. 2020;18:428.
16. Mohanty H, Banerjee D. An Analysis of Protection of Children from Sexual Offences Act, 2012 (POCSO ACT). Available at SSRN 3768096. 2021.
17. Anchan V, Janardhana N, Kommu JV. POCSO Act, 2012: consensual sex as a matter of tug of war between developmental need and legal obligation for the adolescents in India. *Indian J Psychol Med*. 2021;43(2):158-162.
18. Moirangthem S, Kumar NC, Math SB. Child sexual abuse: issues & concerns. *Indian J Med Res*. 2015;142(1):1.
19. Seth R, Srivastava RN. Child Sexual Abuse: Management and prevention, and protection of children from Sexual Offences (POCSO) Act. *Indian Pediatr*. 2017;54(11):949-953.
20. Kozlovski M. *A Brief Introduction to the Indian Judicial System and Court Hierarchy* [Online]. Available at: https://law.unimelb.edu.au/__data/assets/pdf_file/0005/3085178/India-Briefing-Paper_final.pdf. Accessed 11 April, 2022.
21. The Central Administrative Tribunal [Online]. Available at: https://catjudgements.nic.in/. Accessed 11 April, 2022.
22. The National Human Rights Commission (NHRC) [Online]. Available at: https://nhrc.nic.in/. Accessed 11 April, 2022.
23. The Bar Council of India [Online]. Available at: http://www.barcouncilofindia.org/about/about-the-legal-profession/legal-education-in-the-united-kingdom/. Accessed 11 April, 2022.
24. The Indian Judicial System A Historical Survey [Online]. Available at: https://www.allahabadhighcourt.in/event/TheIndianJudicialSystem_SSDhavan.pdf. Accessed 11 April, 2022.
25. Ministry of Law & Justice, Government of India [Online]. Available at: https://lawmin.gov.in/. Accessed 11 April, 2022.

APPENDIX

Answers to Multiple Choice Questions

Chapter 1

1. d, 2. d, 3. c, 4. b, 5. a

Chapter 2

1. a, 2. c, 3. a, 4. a, 5. a

Chapter 3

1. c, 2. a, 3. a, 4. d, 5. b

Chapter 4

1. a, 2. b, 3. a, 4. d, 5. a

Chapter 5

1. a, 2. c, 3. b, 4. d, 5. a, 6. c

GLOSSARY

Accused: This is an individual charged with a violation/breach of the law for which the person is legally responsible and if condemned then to be punished.

Algor mortis: This is the cooling of the body after death.

Autopsy: This is scientific dissection of the dead body.

Civil law: It deals with the disputes related to the violation of the fundamental rights of a citizen.

Complaint: Any verbal or written charge against a person, either stranger or known, who has committed an offense. The charge is made to a magistrate, with the objective of seeking action under the code of law, but does not include a police report.

Constitution of India: This is a document that provides a framework for the fundamental political code, structure, procedures, powers and duties of government institutions and fundamental rights, directive principles and the duties of citizens.

Criminal law: It deals with the legal proceedings related to the crime committed by any citizen of India.

Customary law: The customary laws are the information regarding the customs and traditional practices observed in a particular community or society.

District court: These are established by the state governments of India for every district.

Forensic nurse: A registered nurse who has undergone training in forensic nursing.

Forensic nursing: This is a specialized area of nursing practice that involves the application of nursing principles to handle certain forensic situations such as trauma, domestic violence, sexual assault and drug abuse.

Forensic pathology: Studying the forensic aspects of anatomical and functional changes including the blood and body fluids analysis.

Forensic odontology: Studying the forensic aspects of teeth and biting marks.

Forensic toxicology: Studying the forensic aspects of alcohol and drugs.

High court: This is the highest court in a state or union territory in India.

Incest: Sexual abuse by a family member.

Indian Penal Code (IPC): It is the official criminal code of India. It is a comprehensive code consisting of 511 sections intended to cover all substantive aspects of criminal law.

Inquest: Legal or judicial inquiry to ascertain a matter of fact.

Investigation: This is steered by an officer from the police department or by a person (not the magistrate himself or herself) assigned by the magistrate and comprises all the reports about this specific Code for the congregation of evidence/proofs.

Judicial decisions: The judicial opinion is a form of legal opinion written by a judge or a judicial panel in the course of resolving a legal dispute.

Judicial proceeding: This consists of any proceeding in the progression of which evidence is or may be lawfully considered on oath.

Livor mortis: This is the purplish-red discoloration of the body after death due to the pooling of blood in the vascular system.

Offense: This is an act or lapse which is punishable by any law for the time being in force.

Perpetrator: A person who carries out a harmful, illegal or immoral act.

POCSO Act 2012: The Prevention of Children from Sexual Offences Act came into existence on 19 June 2012 in India. It is a gender-neutral Act and applies to individuals younger than 18 years of to protect children from offenses of sexual assault and sexual harassment.

Preventive detention: This implies the custody of a person without any trial in circumstances where the evidence provided to the authority is scarce to justify legal custody or to defend the conviction of the detenue by lawful evidence, but still may be satisfactory to validate the detention.

Rigor mortis: This is the stiffening of the body due to biochemical changes in muscles after death.
Statutes: These are the written laws enacted by the Parliament or state legislatures.
Supreme Court: This is the apex court and the highest judicial tribunal and the last appellate court in India.
Victim: An individual who has suffered harm or injury of any kind, instigated by cause of the act or lapse for which the accused person has been charged.

INDEX